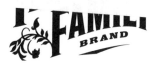

HEALING HERBS
OF HOME AND HEARTH

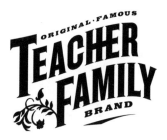

ORIGINAL · FAMOUS

Teacher Family

BRAND

HEALING HERBS

OF HOME AND HEARTH

"AGE OLD WISDOM. PROVEN PRODUCTS."

By Anne Marie Wishard

RUNNING PRESS

PHILADELPHIA · LONDON

Printed in China

9 8 7 6 5 4 3 2 1
Digit on the right indicates the number of this printing

Library of Congress Control Number 2003098213

ISBN 0-7624-1838-9

Cover and interior design by Dustin Summers
Project Editor: Deborah Grandinetti
Copy Editor: Carole Verona
Typography: Granjon

This book may be ordered by mail from the publisher.
Please include $1.00 for postage and handling.
But try your bookstore first!

Running Press Book Publishers
125 South Twenty-second Street
Philadelphia, Pennsylvania 19103-4399

Visit us on the web!
www.runningpress.com

GETTING STARTED

Introduction

Editor's Note: Much of the material in this book was originally published in *Sweet Annie's Healing Herbs*, a book master herbalist Ann Marie Wishard self-published in 1993. I bought a copy of it years ago, and have used it so often, the pages of my copy are dog-eared. I can attest that the formulas Annie provides do work. I know that you will enjoy them.

When Running Press decided to resurrect its Original Teacher's brand, and to publish a convenient pocket guide to herbs, I knew Annie was the kind of expert who could provide you with "age-old wisdom; proven products." She has been practicing her craft for more than four decades and has her own herb crafting business. She graciously agreed to up-date the information in her original book so we could offer it to you in this convenient pocket-book sized format.

Annie's story is below. To learn more about her company, look to her web site: www.sweetannie.com.

My Journey as an Herbalist

When folks ask, "What got you started in herbs?," I say, "moving to the country and wanting to know what to do with all those weeds." It was so much more: my interest in astrology, folklore, and the past; the spiritual connection we all have with the earth; the Native Americans; the magic of plants and common-sense uses. After 33 years, it is still difficult to put into words. It's always hard to describe why you love something—and I passionately love working with herbs.

The "how" is much easier. I moved to the country in 1969 and felt empowered by my environment. I realized there was a use for every growing thing and felt it was my job to find out what it was. I read, asked questions, and experimented. I spent hours walking in meadows and fields, gathering, and using my harvest to make winter tea, wine, and beautiful wreaths. I wanted to do it all. I started growing herbs and realized that culinary herbs also have healing properties. Nutrition was an important part of the learning process. I became crazed with plant power. It wasn't enough to treat and feed friends and family with herbs. Oh no, I had to open a store!

In 1976, Tusseyville Trading Post and Herb Farm was born. Tusseyville Herb Farm moved to Centre Hall in 1987. I changed the name to Sweet Annie Herbs. Because of the herbal business, my learning accelerated. The need to record and share became a priority.

Thirty-three years since that first trip into the meadow, I am still learning. There are many trips to the fields, to the garden, to our large herbal library, and to you. I've learned from you, the people who have taken control of their environment. This book is the bottom line of the past 33 years. The learning continues.

How to Help Yourself with Herbs

The history of herbal medicine goes back to unknown times. Plants always provided medicine. When modern medicine began isolating plant properties and reproducing them in laboratories, we began to see side effects. This is not to say that modern medicine is "bad," but I suggest we take a second look.

Herbs were the origin of modern medicine. Perhaps we should continue that order— herbs first and modern medicine second. Nutritional and herbal healing will automatically bring preventive medicine into your life. By learning to help yourself with natural things, you'll become aware of how to avoid illness. At the very least, you'll be able to head it off at the pass or take a short cut through illness. This kind of wellness gives us control over our lives. It allows us to feel independent and connected to all living things. Some healing plants are as close as your backyard and some you will find halfway around the world. You don't have to be a rocket scientist to help yourself. Anyone who uses common sense can incorporate natural healing into daily life.

I don't advise you give up your doctor and run through the fields, eating as you go. But I suggest you take responsibility for your health. Never accept medication without asking what and why. In fact, if you look at your environment, you may find what is causing the pain and save an office call. If you discover what caused your illness, you'll find it isn't too difficult to determine what to do about it. Best of all, you can prevent it from recurring.

There are many paths to good health. I suggest you include herbs and nutrition on this trip. Whatever else you do, these will help support emotional and physical health. Today, many physicians recognize the importance of herbs and nutrition. As a result, it is easier to combine old remedies with modern medicine to improve quality of life.

THE FORMS HERBS CAN TAKE

You can use herbs in many ways—in the bath, in tea, in capsules, as a poultice, or in a tincture. The following are some general ways to prepare your herbal remedy.

Tea: The general rule for making herbal tea is one teaspoon of the dried herbs per cup. If you use fresh herbs, use 2 teaspoons per cup. You can make more than one cup at a time. I usually make a quart or more if I need to drink 2 or more cups per day. You can refrigerate your tea or leave it safely on the counter for a day. When making a cup of tea with flowers and leaves, pour boiling water over the herbs, cover, and steep for at least 15 minutes. If you are using a combination of herbs with many seeds, roots or barks, place the herbs in the water and boil. Reduce the heat, cover, and simmer for 20 minutes. Remove from the heat and steep for another 10 minutes. In my opinion, you can't steep herbs too long. For sun tea, use one ounce of herbs per gallon—about ¾ of a cup of herbs. Place the jar in the sun for six hours or more. Adding sweetener to your tea does not change the medicinal value of the herbs.

Capsules: The convenience of using herbs in capsules is obvious. If you travel, work away from home, or just don't like the taste of the herbs, you can take them in capsule form. Not every herb comes in capsule form, so make your own. Grind your dry herbs in a blender or coffee mill. This gives your mixture a better texture and insures proper filling of the capsules. We usually use '00' size capsules. You can easily hand fill these. Pull your capsule apart and fill the large end with the herbs. Put the top on and you've got it! Two '00' capsules equal one strong cup of tea.

Please note: When using blood purifiers and when trying to stimulate the kidneys, it's best to drink your herbs. Also, be sure to drink a glass of water when taking capsules.

Tinctures: The easiest way to make a tincture is to place one to two ounces of herbs into a pint of brandy and seal. Place the mixture in a warm place for two or three weeks. Strain and use. The tincture can be used straight from the bottle or mixed with water.

Salve: To make your own salve or ointment, use a base of lard, olive oil, mineral oil, petrolatum, or glycerin. These can be combined or used alone. The easiest way is to place your base in a pan (like a broiler pan bottom) and warm it in the oven until the base is liquid. Then grind or crush the herbs and place the herbs in the pan with the base. I generally put as many herbs in the pan as will fit. Then, place it back in the oven and turn the heat to about 300 degrees for about one hour.

Every oven is different, so experiment with yours. You don't want to boil the liquid. Remove from the oven, let cool, and strain. Store the salve in a cool place or refrigerate if you have used lard as a base. My favorite herbs for a healing salve are comfrey, chickweed, plantain, golden seal, and aloe. Add a little vitamin E and some zinc, if you have it available.

Infusion: Take one and a half ounces of dried herbs and place in a pan. Add one quart of cold water and bring to a boil. Remove from the heat and let cool to room temperature. Strain and press juices from the herbs into a quart jar. Add enough water to bring to quart capacity.

Decoction: Place 1½ ounces of the ground, dried herb in a pan with one quart of cold water. Place a lid on the pan and boil for 15 minutes. Remove from the heat and strain. Press juices out of herbs and add enough cold water to the decoction to make a quart of liquid. This is a temporary extract and should be used in 5 or 6 hours. Make fresh as needed.

Poultice: When making an herbal poultice, it is nice to have fresh herbs, but you can also use dry materials. When using fresh herbs, crush or bruise the leaves and apply to the area where needed. Wrap with plastic or Saran Wrap to hold the herbs in place. This will also help keep the body heat in and release the healing properties of the herbs. When using dried herbs, place the herbs in a bowl and add boiling water to create a paste. Apply and wrap with plastic, cover with a cotton cloth or towel, and leave on for 30 to 60 minutes. Good poultice herbs are comfrey, plantain, chickweed, hops, mugwort. and goldenseal.

Bath: Herb baths are a wonderful way to treat and pamper yourself. Your body will absorb the qualities of herbs through the pores. Babies will have better results because they have tender skin. But even us old toughies will find an herb bath soothing and healing. I recommend this for sore muscles, skin irritations and tension. To make an herb bath, use ½ ounce or ½ cup of dried herbs. Place the herbs in one quart of water, simmer for 15 to 20 minutes, remove from the heat, steep, and add to the bath. Make sure to strain the herbs if you didn't use a muslin bag. Most plumbing won't appreciate the herb bath as much as your body will. This is a wonderful way to relax a baby and help bring sleep. Play with the measurements; it can be stronger.

Aromatherapy: In essential oil form, plants can help soothe, relax, energize, and heal. Our sense of smell develops before any other, and truly helps the rest of the body replenish itself. You can find pure essential oils and use them individually or in combination. Try adding a few drops of lavender to a bath to help heal skin irritations, insomnia, and headache. Eventually, you'll want to incorporate more oils or blend several into a massage blend. For this, use a 'carrier' of olive or jojoba oil. Take a look at my herb descriptions. Typically, the medicinal qualities carry over into aromatherapy. You'll find what true companions these wonderful plants can become.

A List of Terms Useful in Herb Pharmacology

Adaptogen: Maintains health by increasing the body's ability to adapt to stress and environment.

Alterative: Promotes favorable changes in the body allowing the return to normal body function.

Analgesic: Relieves pain with slowing functions.

Antibiotic: Prevents the growth of viral and bacterial infections.

Anti-cancer: Slows or prevents the growth of cancer cells.

Anti-oxidant: Prevents oxidation; anti-aging and anti-cancer.

Antiseptic: Helps prevent bacterial infection.

Antispasmodic: Eases spasms, rigidity, and convulsions in muscles.

Aphrodisiac: Promotes sexual desire and all those loving feelings.

Appetizer: Sharpens the appetite.

Anti-pyretic: Cools a fever.

Aromatic: A plant or substance with a fragrant smell.

Astringent: Cosmetic cleansing and shrinking of the pores. A substance that shrinks tissue.

Calmative: Quiets and nourishes the nervous system.

Carminative: Expels gas.

Catarrh: Inflammation of the mucous membrane; congestion in the air passages.

Cathartic: A strong laxative that purges the bowel.

Cholagogue: Stimulates the flow of bile from the gallbladder.

Demulcent: Coats and reduces internal or external irritation.

Diaphoretic: Promotes sweating; helpful with fever.

Diuretic: Promotes the formation and the release of urine.

Emetic: Causes vomiting.

Emmenagogue: Promotes the flow of normal menstrual blood.

Emollient: Soothes, softens and protects the skin.

Expectorant: Expels mucus from the respiratory tract.

Febrifuge: Reduces and dispels fevers.

Fungicide: Kills fungus.

Galactagogue: Promotes quality breast milk.

Hepatic: Supports and nourishes the liver.

Hemostatic: Controls or stops bleeding.

Laxative: Mild promotion of bowel evacuation.

Nervine: Soothes, nourishes, and restores the nervous system.

Purgative: Promotes drastic bowel evacuation.

Refrigerant: Cooling.

Restorative: Something that brings a person back to normal and good health.

Relaxant: Lessen tension and pain without sedation.

Sedative: Slows activity and helps to relax.

Stimulant: Speeds up activity; often past one's normal limit.

Tonic: Nourishing to the function of muscles, organs and systems. Generally improves health.

Vermifuge: Expels worms from the intestines.

Vulnerary: To be used for the healing of wounds.

Recommended Herbs For Various Conditions

Acne: Burdock, echinacea, elder flowers, lemon grass, propolis, red clover, strawberry leaves, zinc.

Alcoholism: Bee pollen, cayenne, golden seal, kudzu, passion flower, quassia, royal jelly, St John's Wort, thyme, valerian.

Anemia: Alfalfa, chickweed, comfrey, dandelion, dulse (seaweed), elecampane, ground ivy, Iceland moss, milfoil, nettle, oatstraw, spinach, thyme, watercress, wild oregon grape, yellow dock.

Antiseptic: Bay, juniper berries, lavender, myrrh, rosemary, thyme.

Aphrodisiac: Celery, damiana, fo-ti-tieng, ginger, guarana, hibiscus, jasmine, lady's mantle, mandrake, sarsaparilla, saw palmetto, valerian, yohimbe bark.

Appetite stimulants: Alfalfa, allspice, anise, black

pepper, caraway, cayenne, chamomile, dandelion, dill, garden thyme, garlic, ginseng, goldenseal, hops, horseradish, mint, mugwort, parsley, rosemary, savory, star anise, sweet marjoram, watercress.

Appetite suppressants: Bee pollen, fennel, guarana, kelp, kola nut.

Arthritis: Alder buckthorn, alfalfa, angelica, black cohosh, boneset, burdock, catnip, cayenne, celery, chamomile, chickweed, comfrey, dandelion, devil's claw, ephedra, feverfew, hops, horseradish, hyssop, licorice root, life everlasting, nettles, oregano, parsley, sage, sarsaparilla, Siberian ginseng, teaberry, white willow.

Asthma: Asafetida, black malva, blue vervain, coltsfoot, comfrey, elecampane, ephedra, eucalyptus, fennel seed, fragrant valerian, horehound, hyssop, Icelandic moss, juniper berries, lobelia, lovage, mullein, nettles, peppermint, wild black cherry, yerba santa.

Bad breath *(halitosis)*: Bee pollen, apple, caraway, dill, goldenseal, myrrh, parsley, rosemary, sage.

Bed wetting: Agrimony, buchu, corn silk, cubeb berries, damiana, fennel, honey, hops, parsley, rose hips, Siberian ginseng, thyme.

Bleeding *(internal)*: Chickweed, comfrey, ginseng, goldenseal, nettle, plantain, sumac, willow, white oak, yarrow.

Blood pressure *(high)*: Black cohosh, blue ver vain, blueberry leaves, garlic, hawthorn, parsley, scullcap. Look under diuretics for additional help.

Blood pressure *(low)*: Anise, hawthorn, licorice, ma-huang.

Blood purifiers: Burdock, dandelion, echinacea, elder, garlic, golden seal, nettles, red clover, sarsa-parilla.

Bronchitis: Anise, chickweed, coltsfoot, common

mullein, cubeb, elecampane, eucalyptus, fennel, goldenseal, horehound, mother of thyme, sage, slippery elm, sweet marjoram.

Bruises: Calendula, comfrey, garden violet, hyssop, hops, mugwort, plantain, St. John's Wort, willow, witch hazel, vitamin C.

Burns: Aloe, chickweed, comfrey, elder, lavender, plantain, witch hazel.

Childbirth (*easing*): Black cohosh, blue cohosh, evening primrose, lady's mantle, raspberry, squaw vine.

Colds: Balm, blue vervain, boneset, catnip, chamomile, coltsfoot, echinacea, feverfew, ground ivy, hibiscus, horehound, hyssop, lemon, licorice, lobelia, ma-haung, milfoil, mullein, pennyroyal, peppermint, propolis, rose hips, sage, sarsaparilla, vitamin C, wild cherry, wintergreen,.

Colic: Anise seed, catnip, chamomile, comfrey, dill, fennel.

Colitis: Aloe, bee pollen, catnip, chamomile, comfrey, mullein, red raspberry, slippery elm, and remember anti-inflammatory herbs.

Constipation: Aloe, anise, blue malva, buckthorn bark, cascara sagrada, goldenseal, licorice, mallow, senna, wild Oregon grape.

Coughs: Blue vervain, coltsfoot, elecampane, flax, honey, horehound, hyssop, Icelandic moss, lemon, licorice, lobelia, mullein, sage, slippery elm, thyme, wild cherry, yerba santa.

Cramps: Anise, balm, calendula, caraway, cayenne, chamomile, cramp bark, dill, fennel, lavender, marjoram, milfoil (yarrow), penny royal, peppermint, rosemary, savory, thyme, valerian. For continued muscle cramps check your potassium level.

Dandruff: Chamomile, English ivy, evening primose (internally), lemon grass, parsley, rosemary, sage, willow.

Demulcent: Borage, coltsfoot, comfrey, egg white, flaxseed, honey, licorice, marshmallow root, slippery elm.

Diabetes: American ginseng, bilberry, blueberry leaves, chicory, dandelion, fenugreek, milfoil (yarrow), nettle, saw palmetto, sumac, red raspberry, wintergreen.

Diarrhea: Acidophilus, barberry, betony, black berry, black cherry, black currant, calendula, catnip, coltsfoot, comfrey, garlic, ground ivy, hyssop, mullein, peppermint, red raspberry leaves, sage, savory, slippery elm, thyme.

Digestion: Acidophilus capsules, catnip, chamomile, lovage, marjoram, mint, parsley, rosemary, sage, slippery elm, savory.

Diuretic: Alfalfa, bladder wrack, buchu leaves, chamomile, chicory, chickweed, comfrey, cornsilk, cubeb, dandelion, elder flower, hyssop, parsley, peppermint, raspberry, sassafras, teaberry, uva ursi.

Dizziness: Balm, betony, catnip, hawthorn, lavender, motherwort, sage, peppermint.

Douche: Barberry bark, calendula, comfrey, garlic, goldenseal, juniper berries, myrrh, pau d' arco, rosemary, sage, slippery elm.

Emmenagogues: Chamomile, cohosh (black and blue), ground pine, licorice, myrrh, pennyroyal, rue, tansy. Avoid these herbs during pregnancy. Read about individual herbs to determine how to use them.

Expectorant: Acacia, garlic, gum benzoin, hyssop, lobelia, mullein, thyme.

Eyes: Aloe, carrot, celandine, chamomile, elder flower, eyebright, fennel, fenugreek, goldenseal, lemon grass, red clover, savory.

Feet *(to soak, soften, and help with fungus)*: Aloe, bee balm (flowers and leaves), calendula, comfrey, kelp, lavender, pau d' arco, rosemary, sage, thyme.

Fever: Angelica, basil, blue vervain, boneset, calendula, catnip, currant, dandelion, echinacea, elder, feverfew, milfoil, passion flower, pennyroyal, sage, sarsaparilla, sumac, willow, wintergreen.

Fingernails: Bee pollen, caraway, gelatin, horsetail, kelp, nettles, oat straw, sarsaparilla.

Gall bladder: Barberry, burdock, celandine, chicory, dandelion, elecampane, garlic, hepatica, lavender, milfoil (yarrow), mugwort, oat straw, peppermint, rosemary, yellow toad flax.

Gall stones: Alder buckthorn, barberry, cascara sagrada, chicory, dandelion, flax, hyssop, marshmallow, parsley, willow, woodruff.

Goiter: Iodine, kelp.

Gout: Alfalfa, buck bean, burdock, celery, comfrey, cranberry, gentian, hyssop, horseradish, kelp, nettle, oat straw, pennyroyal, St. John's Wort, sarsaparilla, sassafras, willow, yerba mate.

Gums *(mostly as a mouthwash for inflammation and bleeding gums)*: Barberry, blackberry, echinacea, goldenseal, myrrh, periwinkle, shave grass, willow, witch hazel, yarrow.

Hair: Caraway seed, horsetail, kelp, nettles, oat straw, rosemary, sarsaparilla, yucca.

Halitosis: Apple, bee pollen, caraway, dill, echinacea, goldenseal, myrrh, parsley, rosemary, sage.

Hardening of the arteries *(arteriosclerosis)*: Cayenne, garlic, hawthorn, olive oil, onion, shave grass, vitamin E.

Headache *(*for migraine)*: Balm, catnip,*chamomile, clove, coltsfoot, elder flowers, fennel, *feverfew, ginger, *hops, *lavender, pennyroyal, peppermint, *primrose, red clover, *rosemary, sage, savory, sweet marjoram, thyme, *valerian, willow, wintergreen, *woodruff.

Heart: American mistletoe, balm, betony, black

cohosh, blue vervain, borage, cayenne, chamomile, coenzyme Q-10, foxglove, garlic, hawthorn, oat straw, onion, valerian.

Hemorrhoids: Aloe, buckthorn, burdock, chamomile, comfrey, elder flowers, goldenseal, horse chestnut seed extract, milfoil (yarrow), mullein, nettle, plantain, witch hazel, yellow toad flax.

Hoarseness (*use as a gargle*): Blackberry, coltsfoot, comfrey, elder flowers, goldenseal, hibiscus, mullein, raspberry, rose hips, sage, slippery elm, salt water, sumac, vinegar.

Impotence, frigidity: Bee pollen, celery, damiana, ginseng, L-arginine, oat straw, royal jelly, sarsaparilla, saw palmetto, vitamin E, yohimbe, zinc.

Indigestion: Angelica, anise, balm, barberry, caraway, catnip, cayenne, chamomile, comfrey, dandelion, dill, fennel, garlic, ginger, horseradish, lavender, lovage, peppermint, sage, slippery elm, savory.

Inflammation: Aloe, black cohosh, chamomile, coltsfoot, comfrey, cucumber, devil's claw, echinacea, evening of primrose, fenugreek, ginseng, goldenseal, mugwort, propolis, sarsaparilla, slippery elm, willow, wintergreen, witch hazel, yucca.

Insect repellents *(for you and your pets)*: Bay, cedarwood, eucalyptus, feverfew, mints, pennyroyal, southernwood, wormwood.

Insomnia: Balm, catnip, calcium, chamomile, comfrey, dill, hawthorn, hops, lavender, passion flower, scullcap, thyme, valerian.

Kidneys: Alfalfa, aloe, celery, chickory, chick weed, cleavers, corn silk, dandelion, hepatica, horsetail, mallow, oat straw, parsley, pipsissewa, rose hips, wild Oregon grape.

Lactation *(to promote milk—*will stop it)*: Anise, basil, *black walnut, caraway, dill, *English walnut, fennel, fenugreek, hops, Icelandic moss, lavender, parsley, red raspberry, *sage.

Liver: Alder buckthorn, barberry, black cohosh, bloodroot, burdock, cascara sagrada, chicory, dandelion, garlic, gentian, hepatica, mandrake, marshmallow, milk thistle extract, oat straw, red clover, rosemary, wild Oregon grape.

Lungs: Blue vervain, coltsfoot, chickweed, comfrey, eucalyptus, fenugreek ground ivy, hyssop, Icelandic moss, Irish moss, milfoil (yarrow), mullein, pennyroyal, propolis, sage, slippery elm.

Menopause: Angelica, bee pollen, black cohosh, blessed thistle, dong quai, evening primrose, hops, lady's mantle, lemon balm, licorice, motherwort, nettles, red clover, red raspberry, royal jelly, sarsaparilla, scullcap, Siberian ginseng, valerian, vitamin E, vitex (chaste tree berry), yellow dock.

Menstruation Cramps: chamomile, cramp bark, hops, pennyroyal, rosemary, sage, thyme. Excessive—comfrey, dong quai, goldenseal, milfoil (yarrow), red raspberry, sarsaparilla.

Late menses— black and blue cohosh, licorice, lovage, pennyroyal, tansy.

Morning sickness: Black raspberry, catnip, cinnamon, comfrey leaves, red clover, red raspberry, yarrow.

Muscle relaxer: Agrimony, burdock, comfrey, hops, lavender, mugwort, valerian, wintergreen.

Nausea: Anise, balm, bee balm, caraway, calendula, catnip, chamomile, clove, comfrey, ginger, goldenseal, hops, lavender, peppermint, raspberry, savory, slippery elm.

Nervous conditions: Asafetida, balm, borage, catnip, chamomile, comfrey, hawthorn, hops, jasmine, lavender, lemon balm, linden, passion flower, scullcap, squaw vine, valerian.

Nightmares: Betony, borage, catnip, chamomile, comfrey, hops, lavender, valerian.

Prostate: Burdock, garlic, goldenseal, nettle, parsley, peppermint, propolis, red clover, saw palmetto, zinc.

Sinus: Blue vervain, coltsfoot, elder flower, garlic, goldenseal, hibiscus, hyssop, mullein, propolis, rose hips, sage, thyme, wild cherry bark, yarrow.

Shingles: B complex, bee pollen, cayenne, L-lysine, propolis, vitamin C, vitamin E, and bathe in any of the skin herbs.

Skin: All heal, aloe, barberry, burdock, calendula, celandine, chamomile, chickweed, comfrey, cucumber, elder, garden violet, goldenseal, herb Robert, lavender, mugwort, mullein, plantain, red clover, rosemary, sage, witch hazel, yellow dock, zinc.

Smoking *(to stop)*: black cohosh, blue vervain, catnip, cinnamon sticks, coltsfoot, echinacea, lavender, licorice root sticks, motherwort, peppermint, quassia, red clover, scullcap, slippery elm, valerian.

Sore throat: Barberry, burdock, comfrey, fenugreek, goldenseal, ground ivy, horehound, hyssop, juniper, lemon , mallow, myrrh, rose hip, sage, salt and vinegar water, savory, slippery elm, strawberry, sumac, white oak, willow, wintergreen, witch hazel.

Stimulants: Caraway, cardamom, coffee, gota kola, guarana, kola nut, ma haung (Chinese ephreda), yerba mate.

Stomach: Alfalfa, balm, burdock, calendula, caraway, catnip, cayenne, chamomile, chickweed, chicory, clove, comfrey, fennel, fenugreek, garlic, ginger, hops, Icelandic moss, juniper, lavender, lemon balm, licorice, lovage, milfoil (yarrow), nettle, nutmeg, orange, plantain, sage, savory, shave grass, slippery elm, star anise, sweet flag, thyme.

Tonsillitis: Echinacea, goldenseal, lemon, mallow, mullein, peppermint, propolis , sage, slippery elm, willow, witch hazel.

Toothache: Clove oil, coenzyme Q-10, oregano, peppermint, propolis, yarrow.

Tonic, immune system: Alfalfa, astralagus, dandelion, dong quai, echinacea, ginseng, kelp, sarsaparilla, Siberian ginseng, oatstraw, pau d' arco.

Varicose veins: Barberry, calendula, cayenne, hawthorn, horse chestnut seed extract, horsetail, sassafras, shepherd's purse, white oak bark, witch hazel, vitamin E.

Venereal disease *(sexually transmitted diseases)*: Burdock, cubeb, echinacea, frankincense, goldenseal, juniper, milfoil (yarrow), parsley, pipsissewa, saw palmetto, slippery elm, sumac, wild Oregon grape, witch hazel, yellow dock.

Warts: American ash tree, buckthorn, calendula, celandine, dandelion, garlic, mullein.

Worms: Aloe, black walnut, buck bean, garden thyme, garlic, mugwort, onion, pumpkin seeds, quassia, senna, southernwood, tansy, white oak, wormwood.

Wounds: Aloe, amaranth, arnica, blackberry, calendula, chamomile, chickweed, cleavers, comfrey, dandelion, echinacea, flax, gentian, goldenseal, lady's mantle, onion, plantain, St. John's Wort, shave grass, slippery elm, willow, yellow bedstraw.

GLOSSARY OF HEALING HERBS

FROM ALOE TO YOHIMBE: PERTINENT FACTS
ABOUT THE MOST POTENT HERBS

ALOE *(Aloe vera):*

A member of the lily family, aloe grows naturally in warmer climates. For those who live in the north, it is easy to grow as a houseplant. The older plants (3 years or more) produce the most healing juice. The juice has a gel-like consistency, making it is easy to apply. Aloe is used as a body cleanser (laxative) and a blood purifier. It is emollient, purgative and vulnerary. It's most often used for abrasions, burns and cold sores, and as a skin moisturizer and under-arm deodorant. It can also be used as a soothing eye drop. We put aloe powder in our herb baths for healing and moisturizing. Try using 2 parts water to 1 part gel for a hair setting lotion.

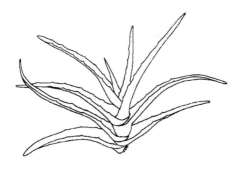

ALFALFA *(Medicago sativa)*:

A perennial plant with much history, alfalfa was mentioned by the Emperor of China in a plant book in 2939 B.C.E. It's most often cultivated for fodder because of its high vitamin content. We use the leaves of this plant in capsules or as tea when working with allergies and arthritis. Alfalfa is a diuretic, detoxifier and tonic. It contains vitamins A, D, K, U, E, B complex, and many important digestive enzymes. Alfalfa also contains minerals like calcium, potassium, magnesium, zinc and more. Don't forget to try the sprouts. They're delicious and full of protein. Alfalfa is sometimes called "buffalo herb" because the big guys love to eat it. Today "cow herb" seems more appropriate.

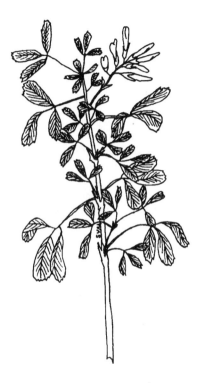

ALFALFA

ANGELICA (*Angelica archangelica*):

This tall biennial is sometimes called the Holy Ghost plant. At one time it was considered a powerful protective plant. The anise-flavored seeds and stock are used to flavor liquors and cakes. The root is the part we use for most medicinal purposes. It is an appetizer, expectorant and carminative. Angelica contains a large number of coumarins, which give this plant antibacterial and anti-fungal qualities. Angelica helps balance the female system and gives aid to arthritis sufferers. If you want to grow your own, start with a seedling plant because the seeds do not store well. Allow the plant to re-seed itself and you will always have angelica in your garden.

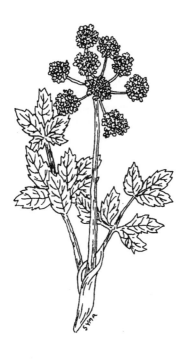

ANGELICA

ANISE *(Pimpinella anisum)*:

An annual plant that has been valued for everything from paying taxes to settling the stomach! In the sixteenth century, it was used for mouse bait. Today it is used in cakes, cookies, and breads. As a medicinal tea it settles the stomach and has antispasmodic qualities. Anise contains vitamins A, B, C and some minerals. Its ability to clear mucus from the body makes it helpful for sinus and other respiratory infections.

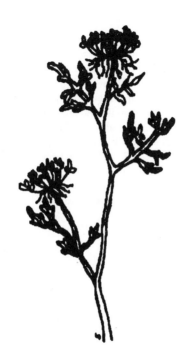

Anise

BASIL *(Ocimum basilicum)*:
Basil, a tender annual, is a joy to grow and use. Old herbals recommend that a naked woman should plant basil seed by the light of the moon. This is another way of saying basil is a sissy and needs very warm weather to do well. It is in the mint family and has dark green leaves and bushy stems. Not usually thought of as medicinal, it can be used as a tea for upset stomach or colds. It does contain vitamins A and C. A good companion for tomatoes in the garden or in the cooking pot. In addition to sweet basil, I recommend lemon and purple basil.

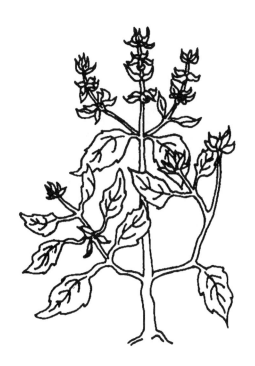

BASIL

BAY *(Laurus nobilis)*:

The sweet bay tree is a tender perennial that originally made its home in the Mediterranean. It can be grown in a large pot and will reach 4 feet in height. It makes a beautiful houseplant. I move my bay tree to the porch or garden in the summer and bring it in for the cold months. I actually decorate mine with small ornaments for the holidays. Besides its culinary uses, bay can be used as a bug repellent herb. It helps keep pests out of flour and pasta. Also, try using it in your favorite flea or moth repellent.

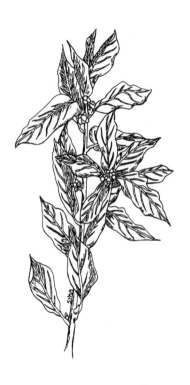

BAY

BERGAMOT *(Monarda didyma)*:

This showy, perennial mint wears a wild red hat most of the summer. There are other varieties of bergamot—pink, white and purple. Red is the one that the hummingbirds, the bees and I love best. An "eating flower," we enjoy it in salads, dips and straight from the plant to our mouths—the tips are sweet like honeysuckle. It dries a dark red, and we use the leaves and flowers in tea. Bergamont, also called "bee balm," contains vitamin A, C, and thymol. It is often used to fight fungus and bacteria. We use it in tea, tinctures, potpourris, and baths.

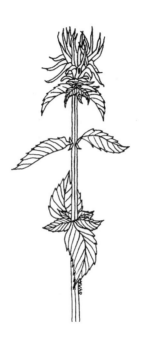

BERGAMOT

BLACK COHOSH *(Cimicifuga racemosa)*:
Sometimes called squawroot, this herb makes its
home in the middle-eastern part of the United States.
Its beautiful flowers grow happily in the woods or
along the roadside. Black cohosh looks like a tall
wand covered with delicate white flowers. Very
magical! We give credit to the Native Americans
for introducing this plant to us. Black cohosh helps
balance the body's hormones. It is an emmenagogue,
nervine and a tonic. Because it contains natural
estrogen, we include black cohosh extract in our
women's formula. It has solicylates that make it
anti-inflammatory. Black cohosh has also been
recommended for lowering blood pressure, helping
arthritis and relieving respiratory problems. Most
often we use this herb in tea or in capsules.

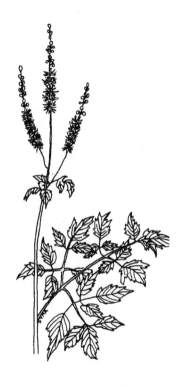

BLACK COHOSH

BLUEBERRY LEAVES *(Valinium myrtillus)*:
The blueberry bush is a hardy perennial. The most
important fact I can share with you is that blueberry
leaf tea when used every day can regulate blood
sugar. It also helps to lower blood pressure. Most folks
who drink one to two cups per day have great success
regulating blood sugar. Recent studies indicate that
blueberries also help regulate blood sugar. In the
past, herbalists have used this herb for kidney and
bladder stones. It seems to have antiseptic qualities.

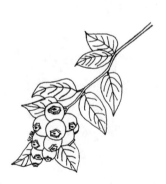

BLUE COHOSH (*Caylophyllum thalictroides*):
Blue cohosh is a perennial plant reaching 1 to 3 feet
in height. The pea-sized fruit is dark blue and berry-
like. The seeds are said to be poisonous. Native
American women drank this tea for a few weeks
before childbirth. They felt it eased the process.
Some practitioners today use this herb to ease
delivery. However, do not use it in the early stages
of pregnancy. Blue cohosh contains the alkaloid
methylcytisine and the glycoside caulosaponin in
addition to other properties. Often used for arthritis
and stomach cramps, it is considered anti-spasmodic,
diaphoretic, emmenagogue, and a uterine tonic.

BONESET *(Eupatorium perfoliatum)*:
The Native Americans used this herb for fevers
and introduced it to the colonists. Boneset is easy to
recognize because of the way its single stem seems
to be threaded through the long, pointed leaves.
The flat, soft white flower is made up of many disc-
shaped flowers. This "tonic" herb has a very bitter
taste, so people got well just thinking about it. It
contains flavonoids, terpenoids, volatile oil, and
resin. Boneset is most often used as a tonic for colds.
Tea is the best way to take it—you might want to
add mint to improve the taste. Large doses may
induce vomiting.

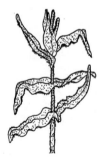

BORAGE (*Borago officinalis*):

Borage is an annual plant that reaches 2 to 3 feet in height. It has coarse leaves and lovely, edible, blue star-shaped flowers. The taste is cool and cucumber-like in flavor; add the leaves and flowers to summer drinks. Ancient herbalists thought the leaves when added to wine made folks merry! And why not? It is a diaphoretic, febrifuge, sedative, and a tonic. Borage contains calcium, potassium, and mineral salts. We use it as a tea, as a garnish, and for herb baths.

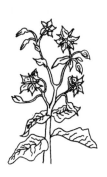

BURDOCK *(Arctium lappa)*:
Burdock is a coarse, branched sturdy plant that produces small bristly flowers. The flowers turn to burrs and hitch a ride on anything that passes by. Burdock is a biannual and we suggest using the root from the first-year plant. During the second year the strength is in the seed. The burdock plant has so much healing help to offer that it is beloved by herbalists. The root is high in chromium, iron, magnesium, vitamin C, potassium, carotenes, calcium, protein, and much more. It is a nutritious tonic for the glandular and immune systems. We use this herb as a powerful blood purifier. It lends help to the urinary tract and the prostate. It is considered diuretic, diaphoretic, a renal tonic, and an alterative. A tea made from the seeds encourages kidney action. We do consider the root the most valuable part of this plant. We roast burdock root and include it in our herb coffee.

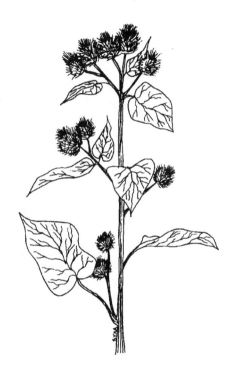

BURDOCK

BURNET *(Sanguisorbsa minor)*:
This hardy perennial has lacy button foliage and
can be grown as a pot herb. It is a culinary herb
that is used in salads and vinegars. Cucumber taste
without the burp. Try a sprig in a summer drink
or in your bath. A cool treat! Burnet does best in a
light soil. The flowers should be picked off when
they appear. Use only the stem and the leaves. If you
are using the leaves for salad, be sure to cut them
young or they may be tough

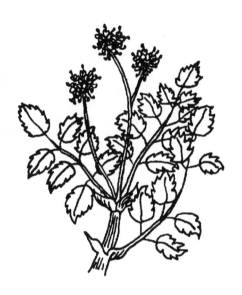

CALENDULA *(Calendula officinalis)*:
This annual plant is healing and delightful to grow. The yellow-to- gold flower can be enjoyed from spring until frost. The daisy-like flower and the leaves are edible. A salty-like flavor makes it a nice addition to salads. Calendula is astringent, vulnerary, anti-spasmodic, and diaphoretic. Historically, calendula goes way back—it was considered the Virgin Mary's favorite flower. Because of that, it is sometimes called "Mary's gold." Calendula is used in salves, teas, and in poultices. We use it for fevers, colds, and in herbal skin preparations.

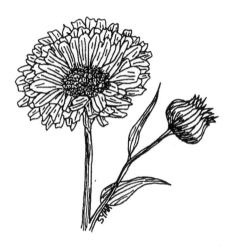

CALENDULA

CARAWAY *(Carum carvi)*:

The seeds of this biennial herb, high in protein, are commonly used for culinary purposes. There was recorded use of caraway seeds over 5000 years ago. Centuries ago they were fed to homing pigeons to bring them home. Women picked up on this and put the seeds in their lovers' pockets. I feed it to my guests in spreads and breads and they all come back. Maybe it does work! The seeds aid in digestion and prevent flatulence. In addition to protein, they contain Vitamin B complex, calcium, potassium, and small amounts of magnesium. This is a small seed so you wouldn't think of it as a vitamin pill. We often use caraway seeds for digestive problems in tea form or by chewing on the seeds.

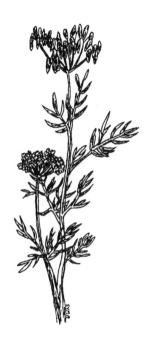

CATNIP *(Nepeta cataria)*:
Catnip is a bushy perennial plant that reaches 2 to 3 feet high. The leaves are downy, heart-shaped, and saw-toothed. The marvelous mint can be harvested many times in one season. There was recorded use of catnip 2000 years ago. It makes your cats crazy but it will help you relax. Cats love this herb so much that it's hard to save some for medicinal purposes. Catnip contains volatile oil, tannins, and vitamins A and C. We use catnip more than any other mint because of its sedative qualities. It's a gentle herb that is safe for babies. Remember it when someone in the family has upset stomach, flu or fever.

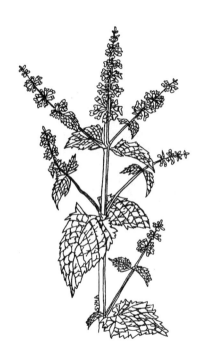

CATNIP

CAYENNE (*Capsicum frutescens*):
Sometimes called red pepper, this perennial is at home in the tropics. This bushy plant reaches 1 to 3 feet in height, and produces a pod that turns various shades of red. Cayenne is a stimulant, appetizer, decongestant, and a digestive. It contains vitamins A and C. Internally, cayenne is a powerful circulatory stimulant. It is used externally in ointments because of counter-irritant qualities (useful for arthritis and shingles). Cayenne cleans the circulatory system so it is useful when treating high blood pressure and poor circulation and for stimulating the heart. If you ever have cold feet in the winter, try cayenne powder between two layers of socks. It warms your feet for hours. We most often use this in food or in capsules.

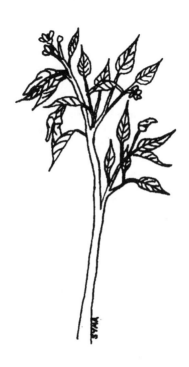

CHAMOMILE *(German-matricaria chamomilla)* or
(Roman anthemis nobilis):
Chamomile is one of the best-known herbs—probably because of Peter Rabbit. The two most common
types of chamomile have feathery foliage and daisy-
like flowers. It is often called "ground apple" because
of its wonderful apple-like smell. The German
chamomile is the taller of the two, reaching 16 inches.
Chamomile, in flower language, means "tread on
me." Because the plant nurtures the soil, it is often
called the plant doctor. It is a calmative, sedative,
antispasmodic, and diaphoretic. Chamomile contains
azulene, a volatile oil. Two of the components—
bisabolol and chamazule—make this plant anti-
inflammatory and anti-spasmodic. It also promotes
the healing of ulcers. We use chamomile (or camo-
mile) as a sedative to calm the nerves and stomach.
The tea tastes wonderful and is very soothing to sip
while reading a good book. Or you may use the
capsules for convenience. We also use chamomile
in skin preparations —baths, salves and facials. As
a hair rinse, it brings out blonde highlights.

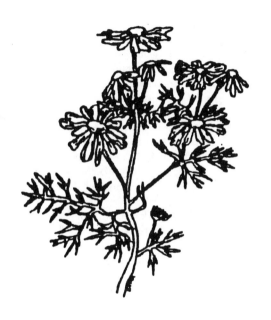

CHAMOMILE

CHAPARRAL *(Larrea divaricata)*:
A natural antibiotic that is safe for internal or external use. Sometimes called creosote bush, this plant makes its home in the southwest. It is alterative, antibiotic, parasiticide, and antiseptic. Internally, it is recommended for bacterial and viral infections. (Cancer is a virus). Chaparral does contain an anti-tumor substance called NDGA (nordihydroguaraetic acid). For this reason, it has traditionally been used to fight cancer. Kidney and bladder infections also respond well to this herb. Because of its bitter taste, chaparral is usually mixed with other herbs. This herb makes a great, effective detox bath. Put the herb in a muslin bag, make "tub tea" as hot as you can stand it, and then soak in it for 20 minutes. Get into bed with cotton sheets and blankets, and sweat it out. Very cleansing!

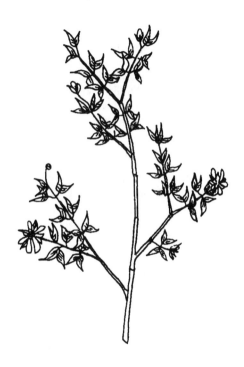

CHICKWEED *(Stellaria media)*:
Sometimes called starwort, this common weed is found all over the world. The name indicates that young chickens love it. High in vitamin C, it makes an excellent salad herb. You'll quickly forgive the fact that it is a garden pest when you learn its medicinal uses. Because it is mineral rich and a diuretic, it is found in many diet formulas. Chickweed is a metabolic balancer and helps regulate the thyroid. As a poultice, it draws out infection and even helps injured eyes. Chickweed contains calcium, chlorophyll, potassium, aluminum, iron, magnesium, vitamin C, protein, carotenes, and more. It is demulcent, emollient, pectoral, refrigerant, and an alterative. This "weed" is a treasure!

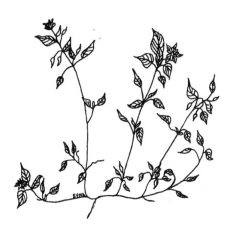

CHICKWEED

CHICORY *(Cichorium intybus)*:
This perennial herb is a common weed in the
United States and Europe. The beautiful blue
flowers can be seen along our roadsides and in fields.
Gathered in the fall, the roots are roasted and used
in coffee and tea. I drink chicory in my personal
coffee blend everyday. This herb is diuretic, laxative
and a good tonic. Chicory helps lower blood sugar
and is used to treat arthritis. We use it most often
because of its diuretic qualities. Chicory is rich in
vitamins A, C, G, B, K, and P.

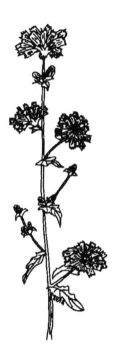

CHICORY

CHIVES *(Allium schoenoprasum)*:
This hardy perennial is most often used as an onion
substitute. We use the fresh green leaves in salads,
soups, vinegars, spreads and butters. The flowers
are a delight to eat. If you can't eat them fast enough,
hang them to dry for winter bouquets. We also enjoy
using garlic chives. Since chives are best used fresh,
grow some in a window pot. You can freeze chives
for winter use. Chives seem to stimulate the appetite
and they contain iron. When using them in hot
dishes, add them at the last minute to insure the
freshest flavor.

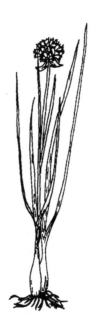

CHIVES

COLTSFOOT *(Fussilago farfara)*:

This perennial herb was brought to this country from Europe. The coltsfoot leaf was often painted on doors to symbolize herbal medicine. If you remember only one thing about coltsfoot, it should be this: It's nature's best herb for the lungs. Commonly called coughwort, early botanists called it "son before father." It confused them because the yellow dandelion-like flower appears in early spring before the leaves. Although the flowers can be eaten, we value this herb for its leaves. Coltsfoot contains minerals such as potassium, sulfur, and calcium. The vitamin C and the mucilage make it a good plant for cough remedies. It is astringent, demulcent, and an expectorant. Coltsfoot is the main ingredient in most herb tobaccos. We most often use this herb in tea. It has a very pleasant taste.

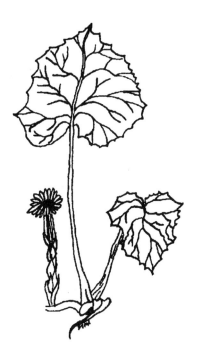

COLTSFOOT

COMFREY *(Symphytum officinale)*:
If I could have only one herb in my garden it would be comfrey. This perennial plant produces long "donkey ear" leaves and pale lavender-blue flowers. The flowers are a delight to eat, but look out for bees. The leaves and the roots are the parts of this plant used for medicinal purposes. Comfrey helps heal ulcers internally and externally. It's also called knitbone because of its remarkable power to heal tissue and bone. The allantoin in the plant promotes the growth of connective tissue, cartilage, and bone. As a result, it is an excellent poultice plant for fractures, bruises, burns, and varicose veins. The controversy around this herb raises doubts about safety. Japanese and Australian research found the presence of pyrrolizidine alkaloids in comfrey. When rats were fed 33 percent of comfrey leaf in their diet some suffered liver cancer. Other research showed that using the whole comfrey plant had the opposite effect. Many folks do use this herb to help fight cancer. As for me, I drink herb coffee everyday that contains comfrey root, chicory root, dandelion root,

and cinnamon. Twenty-five years of doing this makes me very comfortable recommending this herb. We use the leaves and the root. The choice to use this herb is yours. Comfrey contains vitamins B1, B2, C, B12 and E, plus allantoin, iron, manganese, calcium, pantothenic acid, and phosphorus. It is a natural cortizone. Comfrey is a demulcent, vulnerary, pectoral, and astringent. We use it in tea, poultices, and baths.

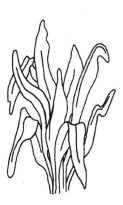

CORN SILK (*Zea mays*):

There is a use for everything, even corn silk. I ignored it for years; when growing up, we always threw it away. We used it for the hair on a cornhusk kitchen witch and then we discovered it was great for bladder and kidney conditions. Corn silk helps with irritation, and removes stones from the kidney, bladder, and prostate. It is an excellent diuretic and a demulcent. It contains calcium, magnesium, manganese, potassium, phosphorus, selenium iron, and zinc. Corn silk is most often used in a tea—alone or with other herbs. Today it is found in herbal combinations for weight loss.

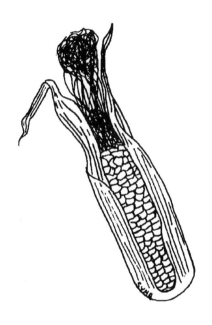

DAMIANA *(Turnera aphrodisiaca)*:
The Latin name says it all! It is a sexual rejuvenator.
If used excessively, damiana tends to over stimulate.
It is a mildly stimulating tonic and a gentle laxative.
It has been suggested for increasing the sperm count
in men and for strengthening the female's egg. It is a
mild laxative, relieves headache, and helps control
bedwetting. This herb may interfere with iron
absorption, so don't use it over long periods of time.
If you're anemic, avoid using it. You can find it in
teas or in capsule form at the health food store

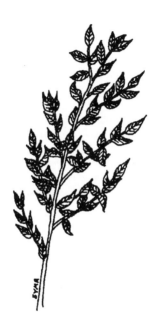

DANDELION *(Taraxacum officinale)*:
Dandelion or "lions teeth" grows all over the world
except in the tropics and in deserts. Some folks feel
that this hated weed dominates the world. Dandelion
is a very useful and neglected plant. You can eat the
new greens, make wine from the flowers, and use the
root for medicinal purposes. The whole plant makes
a natural dye. Dandelion contains iron, manganese,
phosphorus, protein, calcium, chromium, and vitamins A and C. It is a powerful friend to the bladder
and the liver. Dandelion is a blood cleanser that
supports liver function. It improves the function of
the spleen, pancreas, kidneys, and stomach. This
herb is a diuretic, hepatic, aperient, and tonic. We
most often take it as a tea or in capsules.

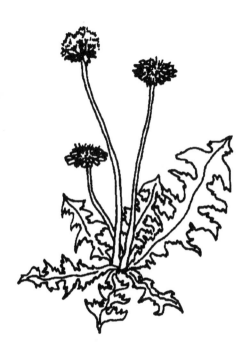

DANDELION

DEVIL'S CLAW *(Harpogophytum procumbens)*:
Originally from Africa, this plant is most often
used for arthritis. Tests have shown that devil's claw
has anti-inflammatory properties. It is diuretic and
seems to stimulate the liver and gall bladder. It is
an alterative and a stimulant. We use it in teas with
other herbs to treat arthritis. As a blood cleanser,
devil's claw will remove deposits from the joints.

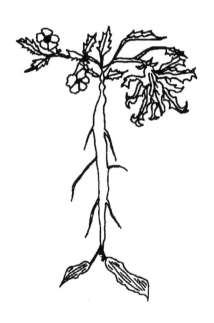

DEVIL'S CLAW

DILL *(Anethum graveolens)*:
An annual herb, dill originated in the Mediterranean.
The name came from the Norse word "dilla," mean-
ing to lull. It does lull the stomach and aid digestion
and is often used for colic. Dill was a magician's herb
and was used to thwart witches. Remember: "trefoil,
johnswort, vervain and dill, hinder witches of their
will." We found that using dill seeds or dill weed in
apple dishes enhances the apple taste.

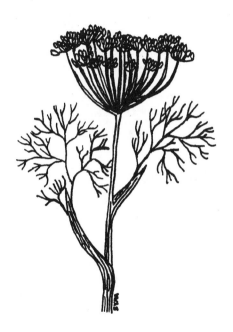

DILL

Donq Quai *(Angelica sinensis)*:

Dong quai is the "queen" of herbs. A woman's herb, dong quai is used to balance the female system. This balancing helps cramps, irregularity, and menopause symptoms. Sometimes called tang kewi, this herb contains B6 and helps with water retention. All in all, it is wonderfully soothing for women. We use this in tea or in capsules.

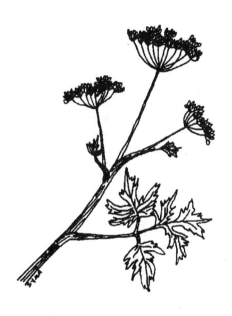

YELLOW DOCK (*Rumex crispus*):
Sometimes called curly dock, this herb is found
all over the country. The root is most often used for
medicinal purposes. It is a good source of vitamin
C and also contains iron. Dock is a blood purifier
and helps with skin eruptions. In fact, it will tone up
the whole system. Dock is good for skin infections,
tumors and for diseases that affect the liver, and
bladder. It is alterative, astringent, laxative, and
nutritive. Put this in tea or in capsules.

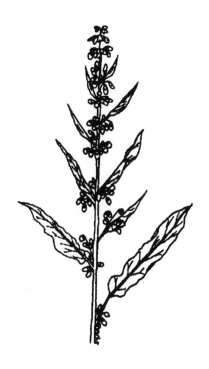

YELLOW DOCK

ECHINACEA *(Echinacea angustifolia)*:
This beautiful purple coneflower is an immune
enhancer that was used and valued by the American
Indian for snakebites and for cleansing and healing
wounds. Internally, it is used for tonsillitis, sinus,
and the digestive tract. Externally . . . for stings,
wounds, and bites. Echinacea is, after all, a natural
antibiotic. More than that, it is supportive of the
immune system. It helps you get well and helps
prevent illness. Research shows that echinacea helps
promote the production of white blood cells, which
fight infection. The root of the plant is the part used.
It is a blood purifier, alterative, antibiotic, antiseptic,
and a tonic. We use it in tea, capsules and tinctures.
Great stuff!

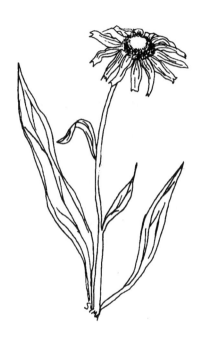

ECHINACEA

ELDER (*Sambucus canadensis*):

The elder bush is quite wonderful and magical. An old spirit named "Mother Elder" resides there, so treat her with respect. When picking part of this herb always ask, "Please, Mother Elder, may I?" Or ignore this advice and take your chances! You can use the leaves and bark, but I use the flowers. Elder flowers are recommended for arthritis, colds, skin problems, and inflammations. They can be used internally or externally. Elder flower contains vitamins C and A, and bioflavonoids. It is a diuretic, an alterative, carminative, diaphoretic, and a stimulant. Elder also helps the immune system. Early clinical trials show that elder has antiviral activity against herpes and HIV. Elderberry extract is effective against the flu and viruses. This doesn't mean you shouldn't get that flu shot. It just means that elder could give you more protection. Elder also has astringent qualities, so we use it in the bath and for facials. Most often, it is used as a tea but the dried flowers can be used like wheat germ. The taste is nutty.

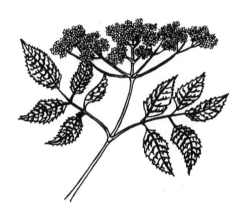

ELECAMPANE *(Inula helenium)*:
 This herb is also called elfdock and horseheal. Elves
were thought to live under its large leaves and it was
also used to treat lung ailments in horses. This is a
perennial plant that grows from Minnesota to North
Carolina and looks like a tall big-leafed yellow daisy.
It is useful for all respiratory problems and for weak
digestion. It is a cholagogue, astringent, diuretic,
expectorant, and a stimulant. It is supportive of the
lungs, stomach and spleen. We use this herb in tea,
capsules and tinctures. Elecampane is said to "excite
the urine" and "loosen the belly." Since it is the root
we use, it must be harvested in the fall.

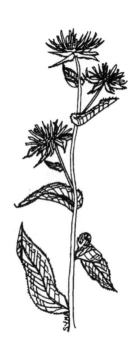

ELECAMPANE

EPHEDRA *(Ephedra vulgaris)* and *(Ephedra sinica)*:
Also known as Mormon tea and ma huang respectively. This herb grows wild in the west and was used by Native Americans for internal bleeding, venereal disease, to purify the blood, and to flush the kidneys. The Chinese variety of ephedra is stronger and contains a form of adrenalin, ephedrine, and nor-epinephrine. This herb is diaphoretic and aids respiration. It is also diuretic, decongestant, astringent, and anti-rheumatic. We use ephedra in blends for asthma and for general lung or respiratory problems. Remember, it is a stimulant. It is often found in tea or capsule form. Ephedra sinica (ma huang) has received much bad press because of misuse. If you have high blood pressure or heart disease, stay away from this herb. The whole herb is safe—it is the extract that can be over-stimulating. I do consider it very good for respiratory problems, but treat it with respect and care.

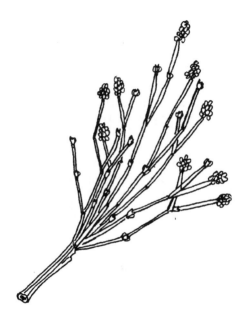

EPHEDRA

EVENING PRIMROSE *(Oenothera biennis)*:
This common plant, often looked upon as a weed,
can be found in most parts of the country. It grows
between 2- and 4-feet tall and features hairy, lance-
shaped leaves. The flowers are lemon yellow with a
similar fragrance. The whole plant is edible and is
used for medicinal purposes. The essential oil from
this plant has proven beneficial for PMS, rheumatoid
arthritis, and hyperactivity in children. It acts as a
balancer for the female system. It lubricates the
joints, hair, and skin for men and women. I take at
least 1300 mgs daily, and so does my dog. Its active
ingredient, gammalinoleic acid, is a powerful anti-
blood-clotter. Most folks use it in the oil form.

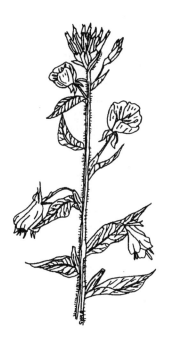

EVENING PRIMROSE

EYEBRIGHT *(Euphrasia officinalis)*:
As the name suggests, this herb is used for eye problems. The leaves and flowers are used as eyewash or taken internally as a tea. Use the whole plant when making tea. Eyebright contains inositol, volatile oils, sulfur, PABA, tannins, and vitamins A, B, C, D and E. It is helpful for hay fever symptoms and colds. It can be used to rinse the mouth when there is inflammation. It is alterative, astringent, cooling to the blood, and helps detoxify the liver.

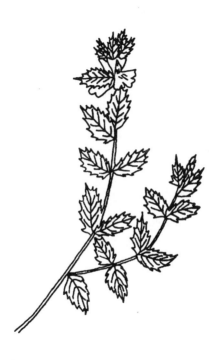

EYEBRIGHT

FENNEL *(Foeniculum vulgare)*:

During the second year, this biennial herb produces an umbel that turns to seeds. The parts of this plant that are used are the feathery foliage, the stock, and the seeds. The foliage is chopped into fish dishes, sauces, soups, and stews. The oil in fennel aids with digestion. The stalk can also be chopped and used in cooking. We love to chew on it to quench thirst. The seeds are also used for culinary purposes. We use the seeds in our Dieter's Delight tea because it is a mild diuretic and appetite suppressant. Fennel also provides a soothing wash for tired eyes. It also promotes the flow of milk for nursing mothers. The seed contains a volatile oil, a fixed oil, and flavonoids. It includes vitamins A and C, and minerals (including potassium and calcium).

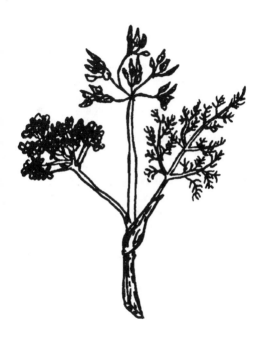

FENNEL

FENUGREEK *(Trigonella foenum-graecum)*:
This annual herb is cultivated for culinary and
medicinal purposes. It is most often used for the
lungs, bronchitis, sore throat, and fevers. Externally,
it is used for skin problems—abscesses, carbuncles,
sores, and boils. Internally, fenugreek is used for
coughs, flatulence, diarrhea, and asthma. Fenugreek
contains steroidal saponins that resemble the body's
own sex hormones. It has always been considered
an aphrodisiac. In China, it is recommended for
impotence and menopause symptoms. Fenugreek
has a reputation for increasing the flow of milk in
nursing mothers. It contains vitamins and minerals—
particularly calcium and many B vitamins. We
most often use this herb in tea and poultices.

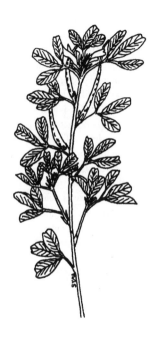

FEVERFEW *(Chrysanthemum parthenium)*:
This pretty perennial flower provides beauty and medicinal usefulness. The flowers resemble a gathering of small white daisies. We use the flowers and leaves for pain—particularly that caused by arthritis and migraine headaches. The leaves are considered the most powerful part of the plant. Research indicates that the sesquiterpene lactones in the plant inhibit the prostaglandins and histamine released during the inflammatory process. This prevents spasms of the blood vessels in the head that trigger migraines. Feverfew contains iron, niacin manganese, potassium, phosphorus, selenium, sodium, zinc, and vitamins A and C. A controlled study in England showed that feverfew used everyday could prevent 75 percent of migraine headaches. We use this herb in our headache tea and in our arthritis blend. When used alone, we recommend capsules because of the bitter taste.

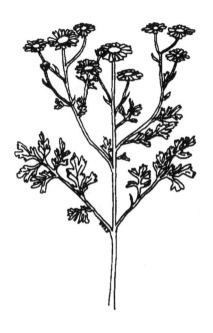

FEVERFEW

GARLIC *(Allium sativum)*:

This perennial is cultivated for culinary and medicinal purposes. The bulbs are gathered in the fall and stored in a cool dry place. We think of garlic as a natural antibiotic and blood purifier. When added to a tea for coughs or a cold, garlic lends a strong healing hand. Garlic oil on a cotton ball, placed in an aching ear, draws out the pain. Garlic also aids digestion, lowers blood pressure, and helps the immune system. More than 200 studies using garlic to fight cancer shows that it does have a positive impact. Its use is associated with reduced rates of cancer in men and women. Japanese researchers found that garlic helps kill cancer cells. Garlic can also be used for worms or intestinal infection. Give a clove of garlic to your pets to help rid them of worms. Add it to their food to make them less attractive to fleas and to improve their general health. Research shows that eating garlic helps lower cholesterol. This wonderful herb should have a place of honor in your kitchen. If you don't like the smell, take it in the form of odorless garlic capsules or with parsley. It has a volatile oil, vitamins A, B, C, and amino acids. Garlic is very supportive.

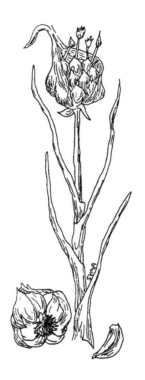

GARLIC

GINGER *(Zingiber officinale)*:
This perennial plant is at home in tropical Asia
and is also grown in Jamaica. The root is medicinal
and culinary. It is stimulating and aids digestion.
Herbalists now use it most often for motion sickness.
It is a preventive and is very effective. Ginger fights
inflammation and stimulates circulation. It also
helps with headache, indigestion, arthritis, muscle
pain, indigestion, and vomiting. It is a carminative,
diaphoretic, and an appetizer. Ginger contains vitamins A, C and B complex, as well as calcium, iron,
phosphorus, sodium, potassium, and magnesium. We
most often use ginger in tea or in capsule form. If you
like hot and spicy, try candied ginger for a treat!

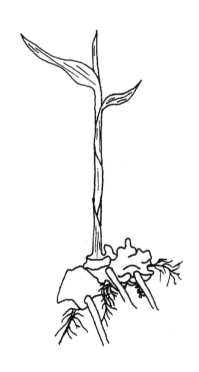

GINKGO *(Ginkgo biloba):*
A very interesting herb that has received a lot of
attention this past decade. It is a powerful antioxidant. It also improves cerebral and peripheral
circulation, so it is used to improve brain function,
including memory and alertness. Clinical studies
show it may slow the progression of Alzheimer's
disease. It also shows promise as a treatment for
vascular-related impotence. We consider ginkgo
one of nature's best aids for tinnitus. This herb is an
adaptogen. Most often, it can be used in a tea or capsule. I would choose the extract form for best results.

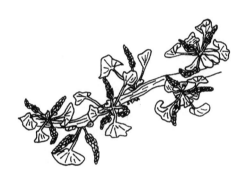

GINSENG *(Panax quinquefolius)*:

American ginseng: This perennial plant is a treasure. It has been the object of many hikes in our eastern mountains. It is similar in appearance to Asiatic ginseng and has the same tonic effects. Often called five fingers, the American crop is frequently exported to Europe and Asia. A highly nutritious herb, ginseng contains calcium, fiber, choline, folate, manganese, magnesium, phosphorus, potassium, zinc, silicon, and vitamins A, B12, E and C. Ginseng is a good immune system herb and is considered an aphrodisiac. It stimulates the gonads and glands (adrenals and pituitary). It seems to have a rejuvenating effect and is good for the endocrine system. It is beneficial for diabetes, lack of energy, and stress. Clinical studies show that taking ginseng before meals helps to regulate blood sugar levels for diabetics and non-diabetics. Slow growing, the best roots are at least 5 years old. We use this herb in tea, tinctures and capsules. In fact, I'm chewing ginseng gum as I write. It seems slightly stimulating and I enjoy the taste.

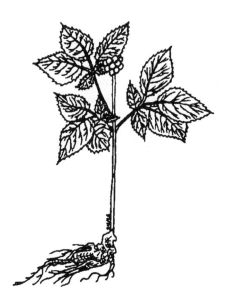

GOLDENSEAL *(Hydrastis canadensis)*:
This valuable perennial herb grows in the
Appalachian Mountains. It is used as an antibiotic
and is a powerful blood purifier. In fact, many people
use it to pass drug tests. The American Indians introduced it to us for internal and external use. It makes
a healing eyewash for injuries, sties, and infections.
For cuts, wounds and abrasions, goldenseal can be
added to Vaseline or comfrey salve to speed healing.
It's a bitter tonic, but wonderful for sore gums and
sore throat. We use it for sinus infections, flu, and
colds to fight infection and inflammation. Most often,
we take it as a capsule because of the bitter taste.
Goldenseal helps digestion and common stomach
ailments. This herb makes an effective douche for
thrush or trichomonas. It contains vitamins B and
C, plus lots of minerals. It is so useful that it's a
must for your herbal medicine chest.

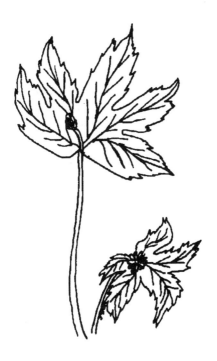

GOLDENSEAL

GUARANA *(Paullinia cupana)*:
Native to Brazil and Argentina, guarana is a stimulating herb that is an appetite suppressant. It is safer than diet pills, but it is caffeine. In fact, it contains three times more than what you find in coffee. It is recommended for headaches and is considered an aphrodisiac. The taste is similar to unsweetened chocolate. We most often use this in teas or in capsules.

HAWTHORN *(Crataegus oxyacantha)*:

Herbalists have used hawthorn berries for centuries to help the heart. Native Americans used it for cardiac problems and to aid circulation. It seems to regulate heart action and is mildly sedative. Studies show that the herb hawthorn helps dilate the blood vessels while reducing cholesterol and blood pressure. When dealing with angina and cholesterol, you should use the herb long enough to make a difference. It sometimes can take 8 weeks or more. Hawthorn also reduces restlessness in children with Attention Deficit Disorder. In China it is valued as a digestive aid. We use hawthorn berries for lowering cholesterol, improving circulation and supporting the heart. We use this herb in tea or capsules. It contains Vitamin C and B complex. The extract is best, and make sure you check the Latin name to be sure you have the most effective hawthorn.

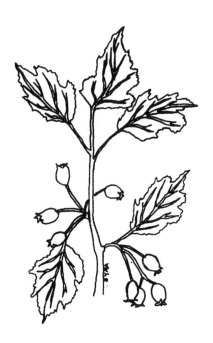

HAWTHORN

HELIOTROPE OR VALERIAN (*Valeriana officinalis*):
This perennial herb is first and foremost a sedative.
It is an excellent remedy for nervous tension, anxiety,
and insomnia. It is a muscle relaxer that leaves the
user able to think clearly. Some studies show that
it is good for palpitations and that it lowers blood
pressure. In some old books it is referred to as
pew—because of its odor. The flower is beautiful
and worships the sun. My mom used to call me a
heliotrope. I didn't know why until years later.
Heliotrope was such a useful herb that Shaker vil-
lages in New England made a living just growing
it. You can take this in tea if you're tough or in
capsules if you're like us!

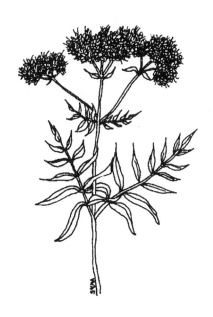

HELIOTROPE

Hops *(Humulus lupulus)*:

This climbing perennial herb is bristly and tough. The flowers are beautiful—so much so that we often place a canopy of this vine over the bed. The cone-shaped pale green flowers remind me of bunches of grapes. This herb is enchanting to some of us but a pest to others because it chokes shrubs and climbs up buildings. Herbal folklore tells us that older women who worked as hops pickers had their menstrual periods return. They also attributed hops for making these workers feel youthful in other ways. Herbalists then began to recommend it for a hormonal balancer and to relieve menopause symptoms. Many years later, it was discovered that hops contained a potent phytoestrogen called prenylnaringenin. Hops are sedative. We add them to tea or put them in sleep pillows. They can be used for excess water retention and uric acid. This herb is diuretic, febrifuge, sedative, and hypnotic. Hops have been used to brew beer for centuries. As a sedative, they're safe, and can be used in tea or capsules.

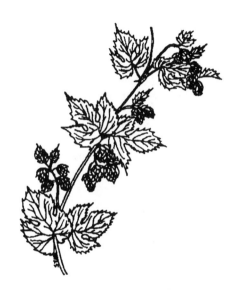

HOREHOUND (*Marrubium vulgare*): This perennial herb was used by the early Greeks to treat lung ailments and sore throat. It softens phlegm, making it easier to expel. Like many herbs, European herbalists introduced this member of the mint family to this country. Horehound is terribly bitter, which explains why the candy made from it became so popular. It was covered with sugar to mask the nasty taste. Once when I had the flu I made horehound candy with brown sugar. I ate it all and felt better. But then, I love brown sugar. We use this herb mixed with others in teas for colds and flu.

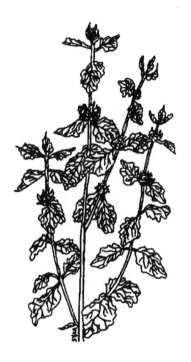

HOREHOUND

HORSERADISH (*Armoracia lapathifolia*):
This perennial culinary herb is used as a condiment and enjoyed for its sharp hot taste. It certainly is a stimulating decongestant. Externally, it's used as an irritant to stimulate blood flow and sometimes it's used in a poultice for rheumatism. Internally, horseradish is used to treat lung problems. Horseradish contains natural estrogen—so if you crave it, perhaps you need it.

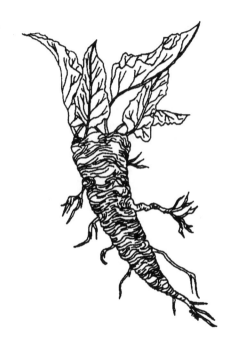

HORSERADISH

HYSSOP *(Hyssopus officinalis)*:

This beautiful dark green perennial herb most often produces blue flowers. The flowers and leaves are used as an expectorant. The plant itself smells a little like skunk. I've learned to like the smell! Studies show that the mold found on this plant is the same mold that produces penicillin. Generally this herb helps to rid the body of mucus. It is used for sore throat, colds, arthritis, and congestion. Hyssop is carminative, astringent, expectorant, and tonic.

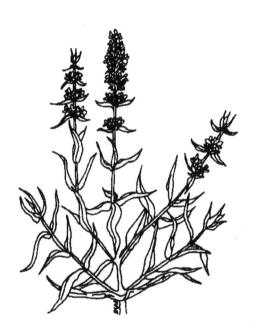

HYSSOP

JUNIPER BERRIES (*Juniperus communis*):
The berries of this evergreen shrub are used for
lung, kidney, and bladder problems. Juniper berries
are anti-inflammatory and are helpful for sinusitis.
They are very high in vitamin C. The berries have
been used to flavor venison and gin. Juniper berry
oil, mixed in water, is used as a scrub to kill bacteria
in the rooms of the sick. Juniper berries are antiscor-
butic, antiseptic, diuretic, and tonic. We use this
herb in tea or in capsules.

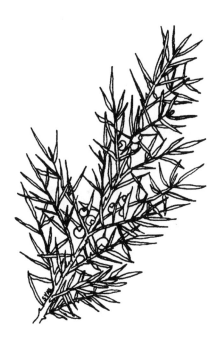

JUNIPER BERRIES

KELP *(Fucus versiculosus)*:

Kelp, the common name for seaweed, contains calcium, iodine, sulfur, and silicon. In fact, it is the highest single source of trace minerals found anywhere. In the orient, kelp is used for health and beauty. It improves your skin, nails, and hair. It is a diuretic so it's used for dieting. We also use it in our herb baths because it increases circulation and attracts moisture to the skin. Kelp, when sprinkled on a loofah sponge and rubbed briskly on the skin, helps break down cellulite. Kelp encourages healthy functioning of the body. It can be used as a salt substitute. This mineral treasure chest also contains carotenes, B complex, C, K, and vitamin E. This is one herb that is worth knowing.

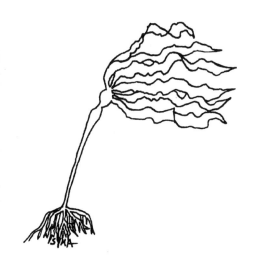

LADY'S MANTLE (*Alchemilla vulgaris*):
A favorite perennial of mine because it is very
beautiful. The leaves are fluted and fan-like, the
flowers are star-shaped and delicate. These magical
flowers dry and are second in beauty only to the
dew touched leaves on a summer morning. The
Latin name for this plant comes from the word
alchemy. Lady's mantle was believed to be magical.
Definitely a lady's herb, it was believed to help sag-
ging breasts. I read once that it was placed in a baby
girl's cradle to insure "proper breast size"—whatever
that means! It is astringent and diuretic, so it is recommended for kidney stones and urinary infections.

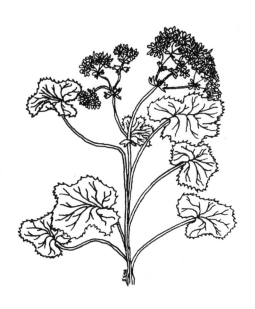

LADY'S MANTLE

LAVENDER *(Lavandula officinalis or Lavandula vera)*:
Another lady's herb, lavender is said to "help with headaches from too much sun or too much house-work." It was also the aroma of domestic virtue. Lavender is such a versatile herb. The tea and essential oil have been used to treat insomnia, fatigue, headaches, muscle spasms, nervousness, and nausea. Another thing to remember about lavender is that it is a bug repellent herb. It is also antibacterial and can help skin problems such as wounds, burns, acne, and eczema. It became a treasured sachet because it kept moths out of the linen closet. Internally, lavender is a sedative, antispasmodic, diuretic, carminative, and a cholagogue. We use the flowers in herb baths; they relax and soothe aching muscles. The leaves and flowers may be used for tea, but we usually use the flowers. Lavender can also be encapsuled. The essential oil of lavender is another great choice for your medicine cupboard.

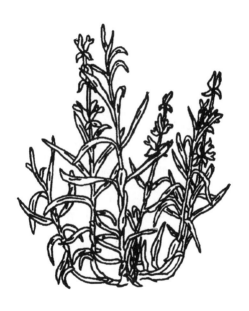

LAVENDER

LEMON BALM *(Melissa officinalis)*:
This perennial herb is one of the firsts to poke its
head through the ground in the spring. It's a member
of the mint family and definitely smells like Lemon
Pledge. It is said, "to be for the stomachs of your poor
sickly neighbors." Lemon balm has helped with irritable bowel spasms. No wonder it helped "those poor
sickly neighbors!" Lemon balm is recommended for
the treatment of fever, colds, and nervous disposition.
It has been shown to help those with Graves' disease.
It contains flavonoids and polyphenolics that help
regulate the thyroid. Clinical studies show that it is
also useful in the treatment of herpes infection.
Because Melissa is an important balancer for the
female system, it's an ingredient in our women's
formula. Lemon balm contains vitamins A and C.
Research shows that it has antiviral properties
effective against cold sores and other viruses. We
use this in tea and capsules.

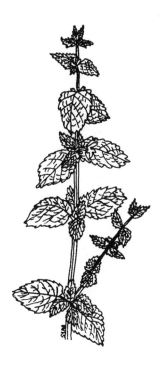

LEMON BALM

LEMON GRASS *(Cymbopogon citratus):*
This tender perennial contains citral, an essential
oil used in perfumery. This is a grass that comes
from east India and makes itself at home in our
southwest. Very high in vitamin A, it is recommended for eye and skin problems. We use this tea
as a hair rinse—it brings the pH balance back and
removes soap film. Use it in tea, in a facial or in
your bath. Lemon grass is also used in Indian cooking. I always bring a big pot of lemon grass into the
house for winter use. The tea tastes like a lemon
vanilla wafer.

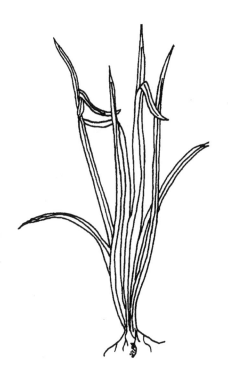

LEMON GRASS

LEMON VERBENA *(Lippia citriodora)*:
This tender native of South America has the
cleanest, purest lemon aroma. Surely it will delight
your nose. Scarlet O'Hara's mother smelled of lemon
verbena. It is still used in soaps and cosmetics today.
Its main oil is citral. We use lemon verbena in baths,
teas, and potpourris. In our country, it will grow to
four feet in a large clay pot. In South America, it
becomes a tree. Although it loses its leaves in the
winter, its fragrance makes it worth the trouble.

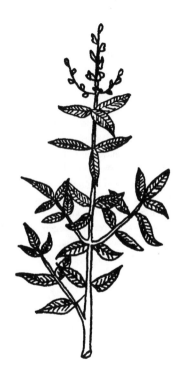

LEMON VERBENA

LICORICE *(Glycyrrhiza glabra)*:
Licorice is a perennial plant that makes its home in central Europe and parts of Asia. It was used for thousands of years to support the heart and the spleen. Licorice root is helpful for many neurological conditions like Bell's Palsy. The woody root is chewed on to soothe a sore throat caused by singing or screaming too much. We could all use this one. In colonial times, people chewed on the root until it frayed, then used it like a toothbrush to clean their teeth. It is still used in modern medicine to flavor bad-tasting medicine, as a laxative, and as a stomach coating. It is diuretic and expectorant. Licorice is a natural source of estrogen, so we include it in our women's formula. Most often, it is used in tea or capsules.

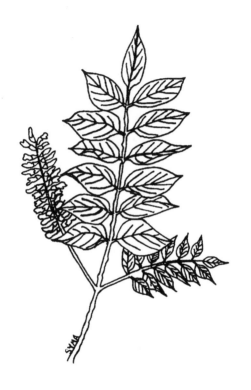

LOBELIA *(Lobelia inflata)*:
This plant, sometimes called Indian tobacco or v omit root, is found in North America in pastures and wastelands. If you ingest too much, it can cause vomiting. Lobelia is a super expectorant and is often used by those with asthma. It is antispasmodic, emetic, and a nervine. Externally, it can be used in a poultice for bruises and bites. It can be very harsh so use sparingly.

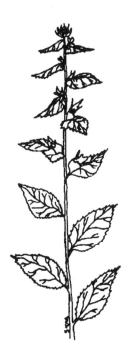

LOBELIA

LOVAGE *(Levisticum officinale)*:
Lovage is not really considered medicinal, but I wouldn't have an herb garden without it. A perennial, lovage looks like a huge celery plant and is a strong celery substitute. The leaves and stalks can be used in cooking. My favorite use is to use the hollow stalks as a natural straw—great with tomato juice or a Bloody Mary. If that isn't medicinal enough, try the roots or the whole herb in a tea as a diuretic. This tea is also recommended for asthmatics. Lovage is an expectorant, carminative, and for a stomachache.

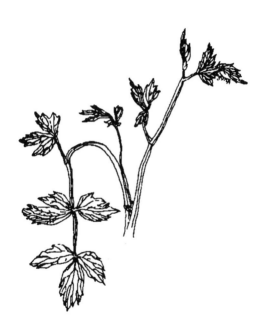

LOVAGE

MANDRAKE *(Podophyllum peltatum)* and
EUROPEAN MANDRAKE *(Mandragora officinarum)*:
American mandrake or May apple loves living in
the woods. The American Indians used the root as
a cathartic and energetic purgative. An overdose
may cause death. It's best just to look at this plant.
European mandrake isn't even related to the
American. Its root resembles a man and some think
it has magical powers. Mandrake root was used as an
anesthetic for surgery. Again, I would caution against
its use because both varieties are considered dangerous.

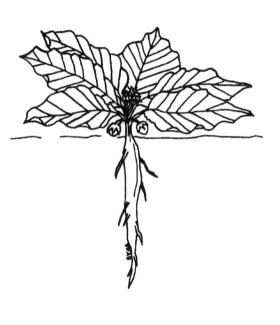

MANDRAKE

MARJORAM, SWEET *(Majorana hortensis)*:
Related to oregano, this herb has a long history
dating back to Greek mythology. The ancients used
it in perfumes, medicines, and as ornamentation.
Culpeper recommended it for cold diseases of the
head. The powder sniffed in the nose was supposed
to "purge the brain." Today's herbalist would use
marjoram for colds and to aid digestion. Marjoram
contains vitamins A, C, and B. This aromatic annual
is great in cooking, potpourris, and tea.

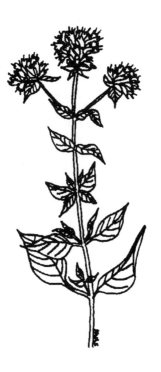

Marjoram

MARSHMALLOW ROOT *(Althea officinalis)*:
Marshmallow is high in mucilage and lubricates.
This lubricating action helps the lungs, kidneys,
and intestines. We recommend it in teas for kidney
treatment, especially to assist in passing stones.
Marshmallow is anti-inflammatory. Mix marshmallow
root powder into your favorite cream and apply
it to breakouts of psoriasis and eczema. It will form
a protective layer on the skin. It is beneficial when
dealing with coughs, laryngitis and even Crohn's
disease. This herb is high in calcium, starch, pectin,
glutinous matter and cellulose. It is a nutritive,
diuretic, emollient and a laxative. We use this herb
in tea and capsules.

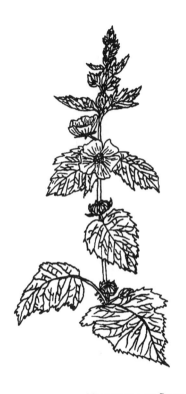

MARSHMALLOW ROOT

MOTHERWORT *(Leonurus cardiaca)*:
Motherwort is a perennial plant that can be found in the northern United States and in Europe. Motherwort strengthens the heart and relaxes the coronary arteries. The flowers and leaves of this plant are used as a nervine and a tonic. It is a tonic for the heart and the uterus. It has been used for menopausal problems, stomach gas, and respiratory problems. We use this herb in a tea alone or mixed with other herbs.

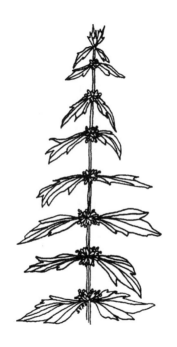

MOTHERWORT

MUGWORT *(Artemisia vulgaris)*:
This perennial herb takes over your garden very
quickly. I first planted it to keep away ghosts,
thunderstorms, and bad luck of any description.
We still grow it in spite of its pesky ways. Mugwort
under your pillow causes strange dreams; over your
head, it stimulates the pituitary gland; under your
bed, great sex. The American Indians used it for
colds, rheumatism, wounds and fever. Today's
herbalist would use it as a poultice for bruises.
Mugwort has also been used to stop excessive
menstrual bleeding. It is antispasmodic, emmenagogue, and a Hemostatic. It can be burned with
sage and cedar to purify the spiritual and physical
environment. This practice, called "smudging,"
does clear the air.

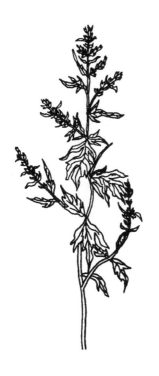

Mugwort

MULLEIN *(Verbascum thapsus)*:
Also called lungwort, this biennial herb can be
found the world over and in this country from
coast to coast. It was brought to this country by the
colonists, jumped from the garden and naturalized
itself. I love this plant and use it for all lung and
sinus problems. Mullein contains mucilage that
coats and soothes. It reduces inflammation and
helps to remove phlegm from the body. At one
time mullein was the only medicine that was used
to relieve tuberculosis. Mullein oil helps with ear-
aches. Its tannins help treat diarrhea. We not only
drink a tea from the leaves, but we also use them in
hot water to steam open the sinuses. It is demulcent,
astringent, emollient and a bactericide. Mullein is
rich in magnesium, potassium, iron, and sulfur.
We use this herb as tea, in baths and in capsules

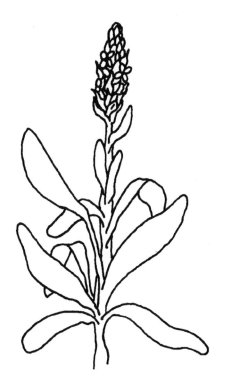

MULLEIN

NETTLE *(Urtica dioica)*:

Stinging nettle is found worldwide. It grows in waste places, gardens and meadows. Once you touch the fresh herb you will understand the common name. It stings and burns the skin. When I was a kid, we called it "burny weed." Once the plant is dry it no longer causes pain. It helps! We use nettle for arthritis, urinary tract problems, diarrhea, healthy hair, and excessive menstrual flow. It is an alterative and nutritive. Nettle is astringent and diuretic. It contains iron, protein, silicon, potassium, chlorophyll, formic acid, magnesium, sulfur, tannin, and vitamins A and C. We use this herb in tea, capsules and hair rinses.

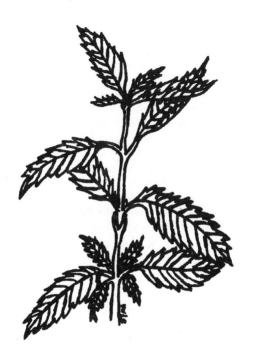

NETTLE

OAT STRAW *(Avena sativa)*:

Oat straw is an annual that is cultivated as an edible grain. The parts used are the fruit and the stem. That old saying, "feeling your oats" gives a hint of what you can expect from this plant. It is a nutritive tonic and a demulcent. Regular use promotes a strong nervous system and a healthy endocrine system. A rejuvenator and considered good for your love life, oat straw is high in potassium, calcium, phosphorus, iron, vitamins E, G, K, A, C, protein, and more. It is good for the immune system and chronic ailments. Internally, we use it in tea and capsules. Externally, it can be use as a poultice for skin inflammations. It is a stimulant, and antispasmodic. This is an excellent herb.

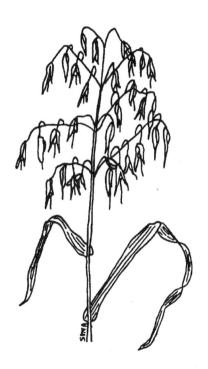

OAT STRAW

OREGANO *(Oreganum vulgare)*:

This perennial herb is commonly thought of as a kitchen seasoning. Oregano was prized by the ancient Greeks as a flavoring and a tonic. It has been recognized for its pain relieving properties. Today we realize this is due to the camphor in its oils. Oregano contains essential oils (thymol, origanene, and carvacrol), tannic acids, resins, bitter principles, and vitamins A and C. The modern herbalist might use this to aid digestion. We most often use this one in cooking—getting the "cure" with the "cause." We use oregano in teas and capsules.

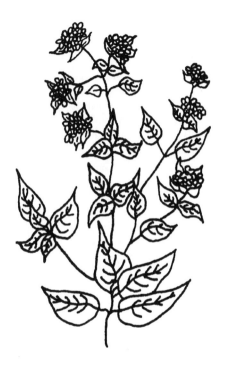

OREGANO

OREGON GRAPE ROOT *(Berberis aquifolium)*:
Oregon grape root is a blood purifier and is recommended for skin diseases. We consider it an anti-
cancer herb. It stimulates the liver, gall bladder
and the thyroid gland. Internally and externally
it fights bacterial infection. Its active chemical is
berberine. It helps treat diarrhea. It is alterative,
antiseptic, laxative and tonic. We use this in teas,
capsules and baths.

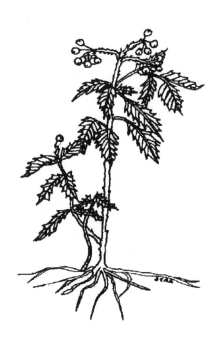

OREGON GRAPE ROOT

PARSLEY *(Petroselinum crispum)*:
Parsley is a biannual plant that is cultivated the
world over. It is culinary and medicinal. The Greeks
crowned their victors with it and the Romans
believed it would protect them from drunkenness.
In England the tea was used for arthritis and to
comfort the stomach. Its diuretic qualities made
it a good choice for kidney problems. It is a breath
freshener and very high in vitamins and minerals.
It contains vitamins A, B, and C, calcium, copper,
iron, and manganese. Parsley is recommended for
edema, bed wetting, fluid retention and thyroid
disorders. The root and the leaves can be used. We
use parsley most often because of its nutritional
and diuretic qualities. It makes a pleasant tea or can
be taken in capsules. It is carminative, expectorant,
nervine and tonic.

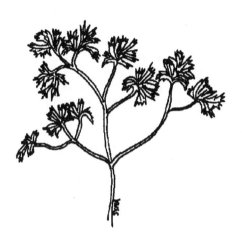

PARSLEY

PASSION FLOWER *(Passiflora incarnata)*:
Passion flower is a vining plant that grows wild in
the southern United States and throughout South
America. It has been used for 200 years to relieve
muscle tension and calm anxiety. It is the source
of the chemical known as chrysin, which helps con-
serve and produce testosterone. Much research is
being done on this chemical. Passion flower contains
small levels of chrysin, so you can feel safe using this
herb. Those small levels are "a good thing." The
flowers and leaves are used. It is antispasmodic,
diaphoretic, and sedative. This herb is recommended
for insomnia and nervous disorders. Some folks use
passion flower as tea, but most often the tincture is
the choice.

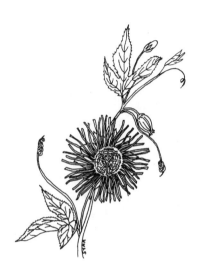

PENNYROYAL *(Mentha pulegium)*:
This is a Native American mint that was once called
squaw mint because it was used for birth control.
Actually it is an abortive in the very early stages of
pregnancy. The tea is not dangerous, but the oil
taken internally is deadly. NEVER ingest the oil, it
can cause death. It is a potent repellant for moths,
fleas and mosquitoes. NEVER put the oil directly
on your pet; you must dilute it with water. Add one-
fourth ounce of oil to a quart of water. Put in a spray
bottle and use on you or your pet. It smells good and
does the job. We also use this herb in a tea for cramps
or for headache. This herb is diaphoretic, emmenagogue, carminative, stimulant and repellent. The
English pennyroyal (Mentha pulegium) has many
of the same properties and it produces beautiful
lavender blue flowers.

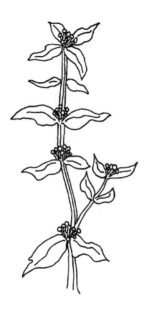

PENNYROYAL

PEPPERMINT *(Mentha piperita)*:
Peppermint, one of the oldest and most common household remedies, is used for upset stomach, indigestion, fevers, colic, dysentery and hysteria. The aroma alone is stimulating and will open the sinuses. Peppermint oil can stop a headache when applied to the temples. In studies in Germany, it was shown to be just as effective as acetaminophen or Tylenol tablets. Peppermint helps cleanse the blood and is supportive of the stomach, intestines and muscles. It contains a volatile oil, menthol, tannic acid, and vitamins A and C. We use peppermint most often in tea or bath.

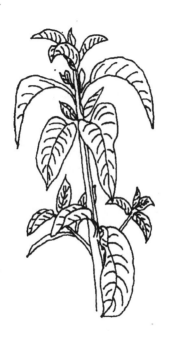

PEPPERMINT

RASPBERRY *(Rubus idaeus)*:
The leaves of this herb make a pleasant, mild,
stimulating tea. It is particularly wonderful for ladies
in waiting. Raspberry leaf tea is recommended for
pregnant woman because it tones and tightens the
uterus. It prevents miscarriage and aids in delivery.
It also promotes milk production. Raspberry leaves
are an astringent tonic to the mucus membranes.
We have used raspberry and mullein in a tea with
acidophilus to stop scours in calves. It helps with
diarrhea in people, too. It also makes a good mouthwash for cankers and sore throat. Raspberry can
also be used in an infusion for wounds and as an
eyewash. It is hemostatic, astringent, mild alterative,
antispasmodic, and stimulant.

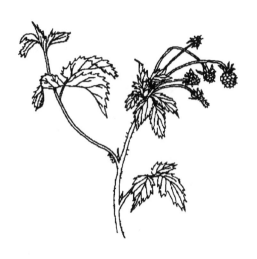

RED CLOVER *(Trifolium pratense)*:

This herb is a wonderful blood purifier. It is recommended to reduce the size of tumors and cysts. It works! Drink three cups or more per day and you'll be amazed at the results. We discovered many years ago that if a person on chemotherapy drinks three cups a day of red clover tea he or she would have very little hair loss and no sick stomach. Spread the word. Even if you don't believe in red clover's ability to reduce the size of tumors, let it help those going the way of mainstream medicine. A fine example of modern medicine and old-time remedies working hand-in-hand to improve the quality of life. In 1996, *The American Journal of Medicine* reported that taking 200 micrograms of selenium daily reduced by 50 perz to be high in selenium. Recent research in England shows that this herb is better than soy for women. It has 10 times the isoflavones as soy, so it is wonderful for PMS, pre-menopause and menopause. We use this herb for all skin problems, internally and externally. It is antispasmodic, alterative, sedative and nutritive. Superstitious? Then, remember "trefoil, vervain, and dill; hinder witches of their will."

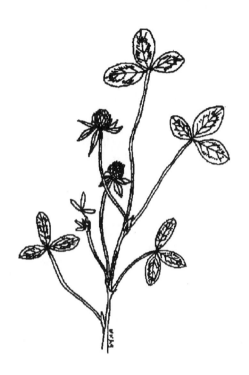

RED CLOVER

Rose (*Rosa rugosa or Rosa multiflora*):

All roses are edible if they haven't been sprayed. During the Second World War vitamin C was discovered in rose hips, which also contain vitamins A and E. Rose petal jam is a favorite around here.

To make the jam, combine a packed cup of rose petals, ¾ cup of water and the juice of one lemon (¼ cup of lemon juice) in your blender. After blending well, add 2 ½ cups of sugar. Blend slowly. Bring ¾ cup of water and one cup of Sure Jell to a boil, stirring constantly for 60 seconds. Add this to the ingredients in the blender and blend. Pour immediately into jelly jars and seal.

It makes about four small jars. Keeps in the fridge for a couple of weeks and in the freezer for one year. The color of your roses will be the color of your jam. Make extra because all your friends will beg for a jar. We use rose hips in tea for colds, flu, and headaches. It is nutritive, aperient, and astringent.

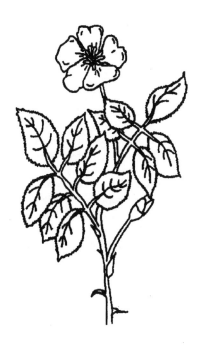

Rose

ROSEMARY *(Rosemarinus officinalis)*:
Rosemary is a tender perennial that symbolizes
friendship and youth. Rosemary improves circulation
to the brain so it's ironic that it was called the herb of
remembrance hundreds of years ago. It is used in
wedding bouquets because it promises a faithful
mate. The name means "dew of the sea" because it
thrived in the Mediterranean. Rosemary promotes
liver function and is a powerful antioxidant. Because
it contains plant cortisone, it is recommended for
pain and inflammation. Rosemary helps with cramping from menstruation or irritable bowel. It can be
used internally and externally. It kills bacteria, so its
oil is often added to scrub water. It is also used in hair
rinses and baths. Rosemary is aromatic, carminative,
stimulant, diaphoretic and astringent.

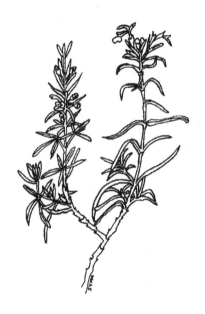

ROSEMARY

RUE *(Ruta graveolens)*:
This herb is the reason we say, "you'll rue the day."
It is extremely bitter and causes some people to break
out in a rash if they just brush against it. It is beautiful, blue-green and lacey. We always have it in the
garden and recommend using it on wreaths or to
keep away all types of evil. It should be rubbed on
your doorstep if you're superstitious. It can be used
internally for stomach problems, nervousness or
dizziness. We don't recommend it internally, but we
do enjoy the beauty of the plant and the folklore.

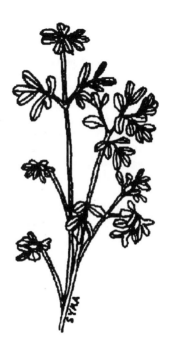

RUE

SAGE *(Salvia officinalis)*:

The word "officinalis" as part of the Latin name of an herb indicates that the plant was on an official list of healing herbs. There was a saying from the middle ages, "how can a man die if he has sage in his garden?" Sage has been credited for many wonderful things—marital bliss and immortality, to name a few. This easy-to-grow herb contains volatile oil, estrogenic substances, salvin, carnosic acid and flavonoids. Sage also contains vitamins A and C. It is recommended for colds, sore throats, flu, and mouth infection. We use it in our arthritis formula because it contains plant cortisone. It aids digestion and is anti-bacterial. This culinary herb has found its way from the kitchen to the medicine cabinet and to your cosmetic table. There are cosmetic companies using sage in face creams because of its estrogenic quality. It is astringent, aromatic, vulnerary and antispasmodic.

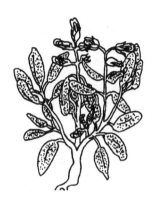

SARSAPARILLA *(Smilax officinalis)*:
Sarsaparilla is a tropical American plant that is
usually thought of as a blood purifier and a tonic.
It is used for rheumatism, liver problems, hot flashes,
excessive uric acid, and skin problems. Externally it
can be used for ringworm, sores, and wounds.
Jamaican and Mexican sarsaparilla is better quality.
Chinese medicine uses sarsaparilla as a diuretic and
an alterative. Sassafras and sarsaparilla are used
together or alone to make root beer. We most often
use this as a tonic herb and for hair growth. It contains a plant form of progesterone and we use it in
our hair tea and women's formula. Because it also
stimulates the production of testosterone, it is in our
men's formula. According to the German E Com-
mission, ingesting prescription drugs simultaneously
with sarsaparilla causes them to be absorbed more
rapidly. It is alterative, carminative and diaphoretic.
We use this herb in tea and capsules.

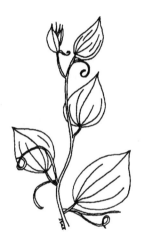

SASSAFRAS *(Sassafras officinale)*:
Sassafras historically has been used as a spring tonic.
It thins the blood, stimulates, and cleans the liver.
The American Indians used this herb to bring down
a fever and to relieve pain. Sassafras has been tested
and found to be a carcinogenic in laboratory animals
when used in large doses. This testing was done by
injecting the strongest property of this herb into the
lab animals. In my opinion, this is unfair testing.
You'll have to decide for yourself whether or not
you use sassafras. We do! It is diuretic, aromatic,
alterative, stimulant and diaphoretic. Safrole is the
active ingredient.

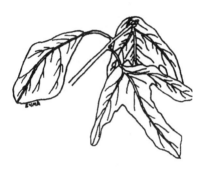

SAW PALMETTO *(Serenoa serrulata)*:
Saw palmetto is a shrubby plant found growing
along the southern Atlantic coast. The berries are
used to treat asthma, colds, and bronchitis. They
improve digestion and are a good tonic. Saw palmetto is valuable for treating ovaries, prostate, testes,
and reproductive organs. It contains an estrogenic
substance, which probably accounts for the fact that
it is considered an aphrodisiac. Some herbalists say
that this herb will enlarge a woman's breasts. I
haven't seen this, but who knows! Saw palmetto is
one of the best herbs for prostate health. It reduces
prostate swelling by regulating hormones. It contains
essential oil, fatty oil, fatty acids, caprylic and lauric
acids, carotene, and tannin. Saw palmetto is diuretic,
expectorant and tonic.

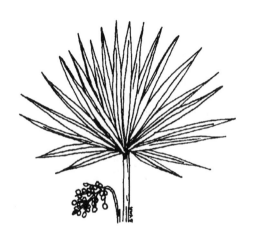

Saw Palmetto

SCULLCAP *(Scutellaria lateriflora)*:

This perennial plant is found all over the United States. The entire plant is considered medicinal. Scullcap is most often used as a sedative. It is anti-spasmodic, diuretic and tonic. We use it in our Sleep Tight tea and in our New Life formula for women. This is safe and excellent for nervous disorders. Scullcap contains iron, zinc, and vitamins C and E. Scullcap shouldn't be stored for long periods of time because it loses its potency.

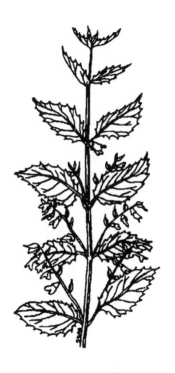

SCULLCAP

SENNA *(Cassia acutifolia; leguminosae)*:
Senna is a potent laxative. The leaves are stronger
than the pods. Overdoses can create laxative depend-
ency. It is not advisable for use when pregnant. This
herb is considered a purgative. Senna should not be
used alone, but in combination with ginger or fennel.
Weuse senna as a primary ingredient in our "Easy
Does It" formula. You will find the recipe on page 277.

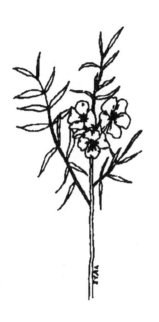

SENNA

SHAVE GRASS (*Equisetum arvense*):
This perennial plant is an ancient member of the horsetail family. When I first moved to the country in 1969, I found horsetail growing in my meadow. I was so excited because I thought these plants were tiny pine trees. That was the beginning of my education. I'm still excited about this herb. It has therapeutic value and makes an abrasive "scouring rush." It is diuretic, vulnerary and hemostatic. Externally, it makes a good wash for ulcers, wounds, sores, and mouth inflammation. Internally, it promotes the coagulation of blood and is cleansing to the kidney. Shave grass promotes healthy hair and nails. It contains silicic acid. Remember silicon is necessary in biological function and is the second most abundant element on earth. Oxygen is number one. Silicon can help heal and regenerate the body, and we are silicon deficient. Shave grass is astringent, antiseptic, tonic, and emmenagogue.

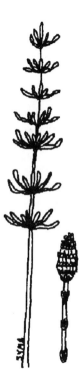

SHAVE GRASS

SHEPHERD'S PURSE *(Capsella bursa-pastoris)*:
Shepherd's purse is a common annual plant that
can be found in every back yard across the country.
It has been used for internal and external bleeding.
Clinical studies today show that shepherd's purse is
anti-inflammatory, reduces blood pressure, and is a
diuretic. It is used for uterine bleeding. It even helps
nosebleeds. It is astringent and is used for hemorrhoids. It will help excessive menstrual bleeding and
bedwetting. It is diuretic, styptic, and a vasoconstric-
tor. It has been used successfully to treat diarrhea.
We use it in salves, tinctures and teas. Related to
mustard, the fresh herb is great in salads.

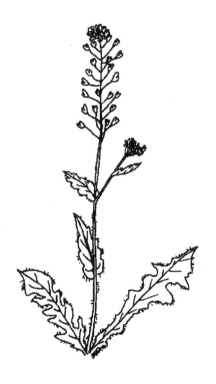

SHEPHERD'S PURSE

SIBERIAN GINSENG (*Eleutherococcus senticosus*):·
My favorite ginseng, and it isn't even a true ginseng!
It is considered an adaptogen because it normalizes
body functions. We use this to give us more
endurance and to treat low vitality. This herb is a
proven stress fighter. It aids the liver and the kidney.
Siberian ginseng is one of the important herbs in
our cancer therapy tea. In Russia, they confirm that
this herb helps to reduce side effects for people
undergoing chemotherapy or radiation. It contains
essential oil, vitamin A, resin, and starch. It promotes
healthy cell growth and supports the immune system.
It helps hormonal health in men and women. We
use it in our "Sport Tea" for arthritis, immune power,
and as a general tonic.

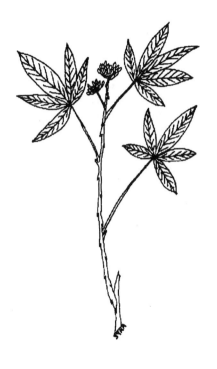

SIBERIAN GINSENG

SLIPPERY ELM *(Ulmus fulva)*:
Slippery elm is a demulcent and an emollient. We
especially recommend it for throat, lungs, digestive
problems, nausea, colitis, ulcers and the colon.
Slippery elm is the Maalox of the herb world because
it helps manage stomach acid. In fact I call this the
herb with a brain, because it heals and soothes any
part of the body it comes in touch with. Top to bottom, it helps heal. Externally it helps heal all types
of sores and ulcers. It contains mucilages and tannins.
It is nutritive astringent, and vulnerary. Add it to
salves and cough medicines. We use it in poultices,
teas, baths, and capsules.

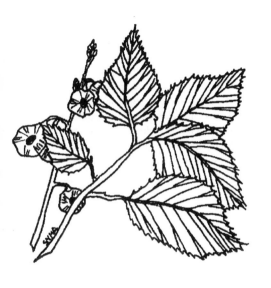

SLIPPERY ELM

SPEARMINT *(Mentha spicata)*:

This herb will always have a special place in my heart because it was the first one I gathered. It contains vitamins A and C. We use this in teas for flavor and to help us relax. Actually, we read that it would control hysteria, so we had several cups each night. My sister Linda and I are still a bit hysterical, but the tea does calm us. It is aromatic, carminative, diaphoretic, antispasmodic and diuretic. Spearmint contains calcium, iron, sulfur, iodine, magnesium, and potassium. I love this as tea and in the bath.

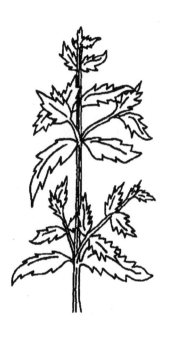

SPEARMINT

St John's Wort *(Hpericum perforatum)*:
This wonderful weed has always had an honored
place in my garden because it blooms on St. John's
Day, June 24. Throughout history, it has been used
for anxiety and depression. Modern science has
proven that this folk medicine really works. In one
open study, 3,250 patients with mild to moderate
depression took St. John's Wort for 30 days. At the
end of the study, 80 percent of them reported little or
no symptoms of depression. A more recent study
indicates that St. John's Wort doesn't work for
serious depression. We knew that! Our ancestors
also used this prolific wild flower for skin problems.
They steeped the leaves and flowers in oil to make a
healing solution. The flowers turn red when steeped
or bruised. The plant's wound-healing ability can be
attributed to its anti-fungal and antibacterial activity.
St John's contains essential oils, glycosides, hypericin,
pseudohpericin, rutin, resins, flavinoids, and tannins.
Folks who are very sensitive to the sun should apply
sun block and wear glasses when using this herb.
To ensure best results, use an encapsuled form of the

extracted herb. It takes 4 to 6 weeks to see results. CAUTION: Do not use this if you are on a prescription antidepressant. Talk to you doctor or pharmacist.

SAVORY, SUMMER *(Satureja hortensis)*:
This herb was called the bean herb in Germany
because it helped to digest the protein in beans without flatulence (gas). It is most often thought of as a
culinary herb but, in our search to find an herb to
help lower cholesterol, we tried summersavory. If
you drink 3 cups of tea made from this herb each
day, your cholesterol can come down 20 to 70 points
in one month. This is one of the herbs in our CHL
formula for cholesterol. (See recipe on page 275.)
Summer savory is an annual that is easy to grow
from seed. Winter savory *(Satureja montana)* is
hardy and has many of the same qualities. However,
we prefer using summer savory because of the taste.
Savory is astringent, stimulant, carminative and,
some say, an aphrodisiac. It contains essential oils
(cymene and carvacrol), resins, tannins, mucilage,
and phenolic substances.

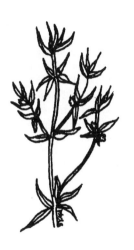

SAVROY, SUMMER

SUMAC, STAGHORN *(Rhus typhina)*:
This plan is sometimes called vinegar or lemonade
tree. The red, sticky berries are the parts used. More
than half of the folks you talk to will believe that
this is poison sumac. Poison sumac has berries that
remain pale green or creamy white. That is the
shrub to stay away from! The red berries of this
sumac are beautiful and safe. They contain large
amounts of vitamin C and make pink lemonade
that is quite good. Try it as a tea or a gargle. We also
use the berry-covered stalks in flower arrangements.

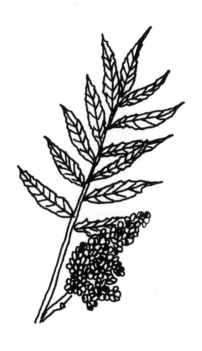

SUMAC, STAGHORN

SWEET WOODRUFF *(Asperula odorata)*:
Sometimes called "master of the woods," this herb
makes a lovely ground cover. Most often you'll find
it in potpourris because it is a fixative. We love the
taste of wine that has been flavored by woodruff.
It is a German custom to drink this wine on the
first of May. Thus the name, "May Wine." We add
strawberries, violets, and champagne with the
woodruff. Woodruff contains coumarin, tannin,
citric acid, and rubichloric acid.

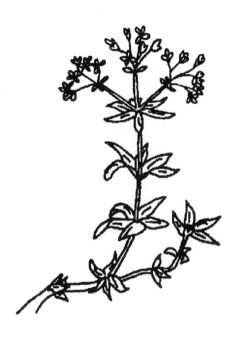

SWEET WOODRUFF

TANSY *(Tanacetum vulgare)*:

Tansy is a hardy perennial that reaches 3 feet in height. Most often used as a repellent herb, tansy makes a great plant to edge a vegetable garden. It spreads like wild fire so be mindful of where you plant it. We dry the flowers for winter bouquets and use the flowers and leaves to keep ants out of the cupboard. To repel moths, mix equal parts of tansy, lavender, southernwood, pennyroyal, patchouli, sandalwood, cedar, and a small amount of wormwood. Great stuff! Tansy is a Passover herb and was used sparingly in cakes during the Easter season. It is very bitter. Tansy can be narcotic in large doses. It helps rid the body of worms. Handle this herb with care because it contains thujone, which is potentially damaging to the nervous system. Tansy contains volatile oil, sesquiterpene lactones, bitter glycosides, pyrethrins, tannin resin, vitamin C, oxalic acid, and citric acid.

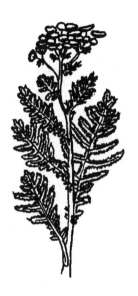

TANSY

TARRAGON *(Artemisia dracunculus)*:
Tarragon is a hardy perennial. French tarragon is preferred. You do not want Russian tarragon in your garden or kitchen. How can you tell the difference because they do look alike? First, you can't plant French tarragon using seed because you actually need part of the root stock. When purchasing it fresh at market, taste it. Take a small leaf and chew it. Now wait 60 seconds. If it bites you back, you will have found "little dragon" or French tarragon. At this point, you can use it in your cooking, in vinegars, and in chicken dishes. It was once used as an aid for toothaches. We never tried this but it might actually work. Tarragon contains essential oil, is diuretic, and can be used fresh or dried.

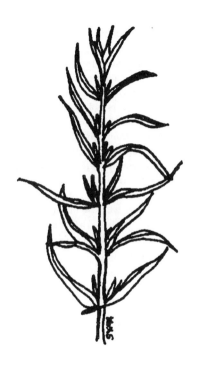

TARRAGON

TEABERRY OR WINTERGREEN (*Gaultheria procumbens*): Teaberry is a common woodland plant with leathery dark green leaves and red berries. We use the leaves of this plant for medicinal purposes. Many folks focus on eating the berries. That's fine, but we prefer the leaves. Teaberry makes a pleasant spicy tasting tea that is slightly stimulating and restorative. When brewing this tea, we recommend simmering the herb for 20 minutes or more. The longer this herb is steeped, the more potent the tea. The essential oil in wintergreen is 99 percent methyl salicylate, which makes the herb antipyretic, diaphoretic, and analgesic. It is a diuretic. So we use it in our "Dieters Delight" tea, on page 00. It also helps with pain from arthritis, so it is in the A & R Formula (on page 285) as well.

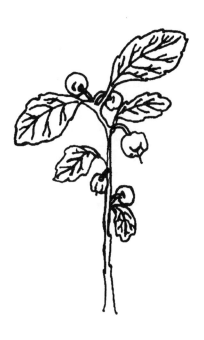

TEABERRY OR WINTERGREEN

Thyme (*Thymus vulgaris*):
Most folks think of thyme just for culinary purposes, but it is wonderful for coughs, colds and congestion. It is an active ingredient in over-the-counter cough remedies and products such as Listerine. Its volatile oil contains thymol and carvacrol, which are anti-bacterial and anti-fungal. Thymol also expels worms. Thyme is an expectorant and soothes the digestive system. We use it in our "Sniffles Away Tea." It has been written that your mate will conquer the world for you if you rub thyme on his or her chest while sleeping. Let us know if this works for you. Thyme is antiseptic, diuretic, expectorant, carminative, and parasiticide. It also contains vitamins A and C. There are about 30 varieties of thyme, including lemon, caraway, silver, oregano-thyme, English, nutmeg and woolly. I prefer the English, German, and lemon thyme for cooking.

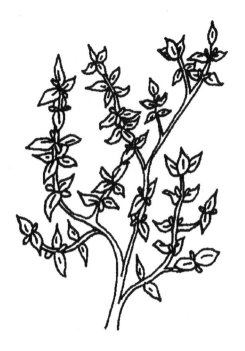

THYME

VERVAIN *(Verbena officinalis)*:

This perennial plant is sometimes called blue vervain. In the Middle Ages, vervain was used in witchcraft and for pledging good faith. It is antipyretic, antispasmodic, diaphoretic, astringent and expectorant. It can be used in tea or in capsules. We use this herb in our "Sniffles Away Tea" (see page 287) because it helps dry up the sinuses. It is also helpful for the flu and nervous stomach.

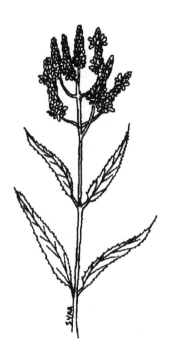

Vervain

VIOLET, COMMON BLUE *(Viola odorata)*:
One of the prettiest eating flowers for your table.
Put it in salads, use as a garnish, and float it in
drinks. Whatever you do, taste it. We love to make
jam from it, using the rose petal jam recipe. The
leaves and the flowers can be used. It is very high in
vitamin C. Because of the vitamin C, beware of
overeating the leaves as they can act as a laxative.
The flowers, leaves, and rhizomes can be used medi-
cinally. It is antipyretic, expectorant and alterative.
It is used to soften lumps and counteract cancer. We
have seen it used in a poultice (just leaves if the
whole plant is scarce) for skin cancer. It is a good
external cancer therapy plant. The leaves contain
vitamin A, and the flower contains vitamin C.

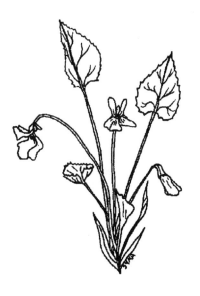

VIOLET, COMMON BLUE

WHITE WILLOW *(Salix alba)*:

The bark is the part used and it's very capable of alleviating pain and reducing fevers. It is our natural alternative to aspirin. The active ingredient is salicin. Because of its antiseptic qualities, it is good in poultices. It can be used as a gargle for sore throat and infected tonsils. White willow bark is antispasmodic, astringent, diaphoretic, diuretic, anodyne, and febrifuge. We use this for headaches. (See page 276.)

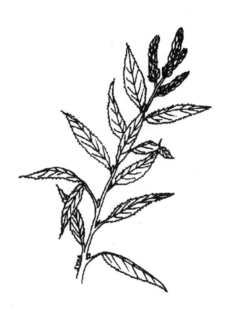

WHITE WILLOW

WILD CARROT *(Daucus carota)*:

Wild carrot or Queen Anne's lace is very common across the United States. I've always insisted that it was named after me. Its beautiful flower dresses up the roadside and the whole plant is edible. The foliage has an anise-carrot flavor, the root core tastes like carrots. In the fall, the flower browns with seeds and begins to look like a bird nest. That is the time to gather the seeds. Pick and rub the seed heads between your hands and let the seeds fall into a paper bag. One teaspoon of the bruised seeds with one cup of boiling water makes a tasty cup of tea. This tea aids digestion and prevents flatulence or gas. It is also considered good for gout and kidney diseases.

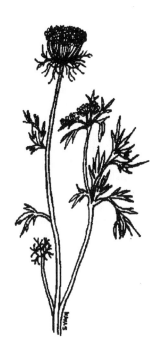

WILD CARROT

WORMWOOD *(Artemisia absinthium)*:
This very bitter perennial looks like a beautiful
silver bush. It reaches 3 to 5 feet in height. We think
of it as a repellant herb for insects and internally it
will rid you of worms. Sometimes called "old
woman," the oil from this herb was used to make
absinthe. Absinthe is addictive, narcotic, and banned
the world over. Absinthe is habit-forming and can
cause hallucinations and delirium. In small doses it
can stimulate digestion and promote sweating.
Externally it can be used for bruises and insect bites.
Southernwood or lad's love is a more appealing
relative. The smell of this lacey, scrubby herb is very
pleasing. We used both of these in our moth repellant. Southernwood is also considered an aphrodisiac.

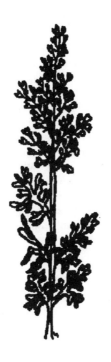

WORMWOOD

Yarrow *(Achillea millefolium)*:
Often called milfoil because of its association with
the military. It was used to stop the bleeding in
wounds and to encourage healing. It can be taken
internally to help stop bleeding. We also recommend
it for colds, flu and sinus congestion. It has a long
magical history. Put it under your pillow and you
will have a vision of your future mate. It's fun but
not too accurate. Yarrow is very good for healing
hemorrhoids and hemorrhages. We use it in our
"Sniffles Away Tea" (see page 287) and in herb baths.
It is antiseptic because of its tannin and essential
oils. Yarrow is anti-inflammatory, diaphoretic,
hemostatic, astringent, and antispasmodic.

YERBA SANTA *(Eriodictyon glutinosum)*:
This South American herb is used for bronchial
congestion. We use this in our "Breathing Easy
Tea" (see page 272) because it dilates the bronchial
tubes. It will also stimulate digestive juices and
improve digestion. The Pomo Indians used this tea
for colds, sore throat, arthritis, headache, diarrhea,
and venereal disease. It is expectorant, astringent,
and stimulant.

YOHIMBE *(Pausinystalia yohimbe)*:
Native to Africa, yohimbe bark gained popularity
because of its effect on the genitals. It is an aphrodisiac for people of both sexes. It contains Yohimbine
hydrochloride. Yohimbine is prescribed by physicians
for treatment of impotence. It increases the blood
flow to the penis. It can raise blood pressure and
create a bit of anxiety. L-Arginine, an amino acid
with good clinical research, improves blood pressure
and helps improve sexual performance. You could
use yohimbie with L-Arginine. Yohimbe is stimulant, antidiuretic, aphrodisiac, and cardiac. Use the
extract as a tincture or in capsules.

YUCCA *(Yucca baccata)*:
This perennial is sometimes called Spanish bayonet.
The whole herb is useful: the flowers are edible, the
fruit is eaten, the plant fiber is used for basketry, and
the roots are used as a detergent. They are great for
washing because of their soapy quality. We use yucca
in our arthritis tea because it is anti-inflammatory.
It can also be used in baths and salves.

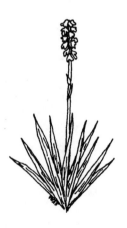

HERB CULTIVATION
AND CRAFT

When I first began working with herbs, I was over-whelmed with the thousands of plants called herbs. It is sometimes easier to work with the ones you grow and gather near home.

If you're serious about healing, it is limiting to set your sights so close to home. So the answer is begin small and think big!

There is no rule that prevents you from using herbs and information from all over the world to create the herbal formula that you need. Information is all you need. Collect books, go to the library, take classes, and use your common sense.

Once I felt comfortable using the plants close to home, it was easy to broaden my horizons. You may never feel the need to do this. After all, most problems can be helped with plants from your own back yard.

PLANTING
In order to harvest, you must first plant that garden. First, decide what to grow. Like me, you'll want to

grow everything. Unless you have unlimited space and time, pick a dozen herbs to start your garden. My first herb garden was a rock garden. How I l oved it! The next year I went crazy and planted a tea garden, a culinary garden, a dye garden, a fragrance garden, and a strawberry circle.

Whether you start growing herbs in a window box or large garden, follow the same general rules. Herbs prefer a well-drained, sunny spot. The drainage is important. Herbs hate to have wet feet. If you have a container garden, put stones or bits of broken clay pots in the bottom of your pots. I prefer a mix of garden dirt and potting soil.

If your herb garden is outdoors, go for the sunny spot. If your soil is like clay, till in some mulch and sand to improve the soil and help drainage. Herbs will thrive with just four or more hours of sun. If you have lots of shade, try mints, sweet woodruff, and comfrey. Herbs make great companion plants for vegetable gardens. So if you don't want to dig up all your grass, plant herbs with the vegetables. A general rule for companion planting is, what works in the cooking pot, works in the garden. An added benefit: the smell of many herbs can deter insects.

Once your plants and seeds are in the ground, weed and water as needed. Fertilizer is not a requirement. Herbs will grow in poor soil. We do fertilize once a year, sometimes more. If you cut and harvest more than once a season, fertilize more than once. We use manure tea or fish emulsion. They both have strong odors, but your plants will be happy. Mulching will help cut down on weeding and watering. Straw or grass clippings look good and work well. Before you know it, you'll be harvesting the rewards.

Collecting Herbs

Many of the plants we talk about in this book can be found in your area or grown in your garden. The gathering of your herbs will help you learn and connect you with the mother of us all—earth.

Whether you've grown the herbs or found them in a field in the next county, morning is the best time to harvest. After the dew is gone, and before the sun is too hot, gather the herbs in large baskets and put them in small bundles held together with rubber bands. Rubber bands are a must, because the herbs shrink as they dry. Take your herbs into the barn, attic, kitchen, or any dry place. It's nice if there is some air movement. In very moist areas, an electric fan is helpful.

How long till dry? Usually, a couple of weeks will complete the process. We didn't mention washing the herbs, because we don't wash them unless they are really dirty or we have some doubt about their environment. Of course, roots must be washed. When your herbs are dry to the touch, strip the leaves or flowers from the stems. Place them in a dark airtight container until you're ready to use them. If you don't have time to strip them, place them in a heavy garbage bag and tie shut. They will wait.

Gather roots in the fall. We dig our roots, scrub them, and cut them into smaller pieces. Place the pieces on a raised screen and put the screen in a warm place. Or you can put the roots on a cookie sheet and dry the roots in the oven. Usually, 200 to 300 degrees for 45 minutes will do it. (Dandelion roots and chicory roots make a great coffee substitute, so we roast them till they are brown). It's okay to get the process started in your oven and complete it in the attic. Store the dry roots in an airtight container. Label everything you harvest.

It's fun to see herbs hanging in the kitchen. So, go ahead, hang cooking herbs where you can reach and use them. It's part of the fun. Even if you don't have time to cook, you can see and smell them.

The shelf life of your herbs is at least one year. If you grow or gather them, it is even longer. Don't forget that you can freeze many of your culinary herbs.

Don't be afraid to experiment with your herbs. Where else can you find something that pleases all your senses and contributes to your health?

THE HERB GARDEN AS A SOURCE OF VITAMINS AND MINERALS

In addition to the herb garden, we will list other sources of vitamins and minerals. This may help you when mixing or using herbs for a particular problem. If you know a person is stressful, use herbs that contain calcium and B vitamins. When coming down with a cold, pick herbs with vitamin C. The vitamins from herbs and the herbs that help change the body functions are keys to success.

VITAMIN A: Vitamin A is not found in plants. Instead, there are carotenes expressed, as vitamin A. Vitamin A received this way cannot be toxic. Improves eyes, skin, mucous membranes and is important for bones and teeth. Parsley, coltsfoot, mints, okra, paprika, violet, chicory greens, dandelion, purslane, curled dock, rose petals and hips, garlic, Icelandic moss, carrots, burdock, nettle, chickweed, oatstraw, kelp, calendula.

B VITAMINS: Necessary for the body's production
of energy. Help relieve stress and depression, support the nervous system, and maintain healthy
skin. Alfalfa, brewer's yeast, bee pollen, watercress,
kelp, dandelion, oatstraw, nettle, wheat germ.
There is little, if any, B12 in plants, although kelp
does contain some B12.

VITAMIN C: A natural antibiotic. Necessary for
the formation of healthy collagen and needed for
bones, teeth, cartilage, skin and capillary walls.
Alfalfa, coltsfoot, hibiscus, chickweed, oat straw,
dandelion, green peppers, mints, comfrey, violets,
ground ivy, oranges, lemons, paprika, parsley, yellow dock, cayenne, wild strawberry leaves,
strawberries, horseradish, boneset, coriander, nas-
turtium leaves, oregano and onions.

VITAMIN D: This vitamin does not occur in
plants. Good sources are fish liver oil, milk (usually fortified with vitamin D), egg yolk and the
sun. Vitamin D is necessary for healthy bones
and teeth.

VITAMIN E: Vitamin E is an antioxidant and protects red blood cells. Excellent for circulation. Whole grains, green leafy vegetables, alfalfa, dandelion, broccoli, spinach, asparagus, sesame seeds, olive oil, sunflower oil, wheat germ, water cress, kelp, oat straw.

VITAMIN K: Helps prevent internal bleeding and promotes proper blood clotting. Alfalfa, green leafy vegetables, shepherd's purse, kelp, nettle, oat straw, cauliflower, tomatoes.

CALCIUM: You have more calcium in your body than any other mineral. It maintains strong bones and teeth. It keeps your heart beating regularly, metabolizes your body's iron, and is a natural sedative. Burdock, chickweed, comfrey, chicory greens, blackstrap molasses, parsley, dandelion, nettles, oat straw, kelp, Irish moss, broccoli, yellow dock, chives, borage, rose hips, horsetail, yellow toadflax, oranges.

COPPER: Important (with iron) for the formation

of hemoglobin in red blood cells and necessary for healthy protein and enzyme formation. Chickweed, nettles, kelp, raisins, nuts, mushrooms, legumes.

IRON: Essential for the formation of red blood cells, disease resistance, and skin tone. Cobalt, copper, manganese, and vitamin C are necessary to assimilate iron. Iron is necessary for the metabolization of B vitamins. Burdock, blackstrap molasses, kelp, sunflower seeds, parsley, purslane, dandelion, endive, brown rice, chickweed, nettles.

MAGNESIUM: Fights stress and depression, helps the cardiovascular system, aids digestion and keeps teeth healthy. Burdock, dandelion, chickweed, kelp, parsley, almonds, dried soybeans, brown rice, prunes, avocados, black pepper, tomatoes, yellow toadflax.

MANGANESE: Necessary for healthy bones. Also fights fatigue, improves memory, and reduces irritability. Bran, burdock, chickweed, dandelion, kelp, green leafy vegetables and wheat germ.

NIACIN: Part of B-complex, niacin is necessary for the nervous system and brain function. Promotes a healthy digestive system. Brewers yeast, bee pollen, alfalfa, fenugreek, kelp, chickweed, dandelion, nettles, parsley, watercress, wheat germ, peas, dates.

PHOSPHORUS: Present in every cell in the body, phosphorus helps growth, provides energy, and promotes healthy gums and teeth. Wheat germs, sunflower seeds, brown rice, kelp, Irish moss, dandelion, yellow dock, purslane, chickweed, garlic, rose hips, burdock, and nettles.

POTASSIUM: Gets oxygen to the brain, reduces blood pressure, and normalizes heart rhythms. Comfrey, chickweed, dandelion, burdock, kelp, borage, parsley, bananas, oranges, paprika, broccoli, sweet potatoes, Irish moss, borage, coltsfoot, fennel, German chamomile, milfoil (yarrow), nettles, mullein, oat straw.

SODIUM: Balances body fluids and is necessary for nerve and muscle functioning. Burdock, dandelion greens, Irish moss, kelp, spinach, bananas, green pepper, watermelon, whole wheat.

ZINC: Oversees the body processes and maintains enzyme systems and cells. Zinc is also important for the reproductive system, immune system, and for the manufacture of protein. Bran, burdock, chideweed, dandelion, nettles, kelp and leafy green vegetables.

THYME TO MIX:
SWEET ANNIE
HERBAL FORMULAS

Now comes the serious business of blending herbs into useful formulas. You can go to the list of conditions and the herbs that will help, or you can use the following recipes. If you decide to mix your own, it's a good idea to use the following guide:

Look at your blend as if it has five parts, even if it has 30 herbs in it. Three parts should be medicinal, one part demulcent, and one part aromatic.

Sometimes you have to limit your recipe to what you have on hand. Don't be afraid to trust just one herb or a simple formula to do the job.

Centuries ago, a healing herb was called a "simple." My first book got its name from the idea that health should be a "simple" or a combination of "simples." My theory was that more was better, especially when dealing with a large number of people. If I used 20 herbs, 5 might work for you, 8 for me, and the last 7 might work for that person we haven't met yet. It's called the shotgun method! When you're working with one person, your formulas can reflect that.

Most of the combinations of herbs I use are based on nutrition and herbs that lessen symptoms. This allows the body to help itself. The most important thing to remember is that "you truly are what you eat." Your physical and emotional health depends on what you put in your body.

Whatever you do, keep a card file on all your blends. You'll never know how important that is until you can't remember what it was that helped someone. Take the time to measure the herbs and record what you do. The following herbal combinations are my own recipes. Years of study and use make them reliable.

When we mix our herb formulas, we mix many pounds at one time. This would be far more than most households would use. So I suggest that you mix this way: The main herbs in each formula are indicated with an asterisk. If you would use one teaspoon of each main herb and ¼ teaspoon of each remaining herb in the recipe, you should have a reasonable amount to work with. This is not the only way to do it, but there should be more of the main herbs in your herb blend. If all the herbs in your formula are main herbs, you might want to try equal parts.

ARTHRITIS AND JOINT PAIN: **A & R Formula**

Alfalfa*, black cohosh*, comfrey plant*, rose hips, nettles, celery seed*, Siberian ginseng*, elder flowers, angelica, sage*, chamomile, hops, dandelion, catnip, licorice root, red clover*, sassafras, rosemary, parsley*, devils claw*, teaberry, feverfew, oregano, boneset, sarsaparilla*, hyssop, ginger, ginkgo biloba, burdock, yucca*, and kelp*.

We've used this formula for more than 17 years. We recommend drinking 2 to 3 cups each day for less pain, swelling and more mobility. This combination of herbs may help after joint surgery or trauma to the spine. The nutrition and anti-inflammatory herbs make it very healing. Propolis (from the bee hive) is also an anti-inflammatory and can be used with the herbs listed above. This formula and propolis can be used with mainstream medicine. Most people find they can decrease or even eliminate prescription drugs after using natural remedies and good nutrition to maintain their health.

ASTHMA AND CONGESTION: **Breathing Easy Formula**

Icelandic moss*, saw palmetto berries*, fennel seed*,

hyssop*, comfrey root* or slippery elm, mullein, peppermint, ephedra*, yerba santa*, juniper berries*, coltsfoot*, and nettle.

Folks using this combination drink three cups per day, or as needed. I've even used it for colds. The taste is pleasant and it opens the lung passages. Asthmatics tell me that using this combination allows them to cut back on the use of inhalers.

Herbs and Help for Cancer

We recommend red clover tea to help a person get through chemotherapy or radiation. It helps prevent nausea and hair loss. We also suggest an herbal formula that we call "Cancer Therapy Tea". The herbs in this tea act as normalizing agents and enhance the immune system. They encourage healthy cell growth. Burdock and red clover are blood purifiers and reduce the size of tumors. They should make up $\frac{1}{3}$ of this formula. The rest of the herbs complete the formula in weight.

Cancer Therapy Tea

Red clover*, burdock*, dandelion root,* Siberian gin-

seng*, slippery elm*, turkey rhubarb root*, pau d'
arco*, suma*, astragalus*.

We recommend drinking a minimum of 3 cups
per day. In addition, nutrition is a major player in
getting well. Stay away from red meat, sugar, satu-
rated fats, salt, white flour, alcohol, and coffee.
Include the following in your diet: grains, seeds, nuts,
wheat and oat bran, broccoli, cabbage, cauliflower,
cantaloupe, carrots, pumpkin, squash, apples, berries,
grapes, chick peas, and plums. These foods help fight
cancer.

To insure that you have the nutrition you need, I
recommend bee pollen. Bee pollen contains 22 amino
acids, 27 minerals, a full range of known vitamins,
and enzymes. Fifty percent of the protein in pollen
are free form amino acids, which are easily assimi-
lated. Pollen contains the B-complex vitamins, C,
D, E, folic acid, and pantothenic acid.

The second substance from the beehive is propolis.
Propolis is a natural antibiotic, effective against bacterial and viral infections. Propolis has been very
successful in fighting cancer. Nothing cures cancer
but these therapies give the body a chance to help

itself. Propolis also helps fight sinus infection, skin breakouts, prostate problems, and inflammation.

I've seen miracles happen with this common sense approach to fighting cancer. Whether it's remission, recovery or extended quality time, these things make a difference.

CHOLESTEROL REDUCTION: **The Cho-less Formula**
  Summer savory*, red clover*, hawthorn berries*, peppermint*, cayenne, garlic and fenugreek.
  Most folks drink 2 to 3 cups a day of this tea or take 2 to 6 capsules. Don't forget that diet and exercise will bring cholesterol down even further.

HAIR HEALTH: to strengthen and increase rate of growth.
  Sarsaparilla*, burdock, nettles*, dandelion, caraway, oat straw, horsetail, kelp.
  Everyone wants beautiful, healthy hair. It's not only attractive; it reflects good health, as well. The herbs that we recommend will not give you more hair, but they will slow down hair loss.
  In many cases, hair loss is caused by stress. To help relieve stress, I recommend adding a good B complex

to the herbs listed below. I prefer bee pollen for stress because it contains the B vitamins and lots of protein. For women experiencing thinning hair related to menopause, I recommend a women's formula. Look for this under menopause in this section.

Remember, hair growth is usually measured ⅛ to ¼ of an inch per month. Drink one to two cups of this combination everyday and you will see more than normal growth. It takes about two months to see a big difference. It really works.

HEADACHE HERBS: **Tension, Migraine or Sinus**

Feverfew leaves and flowers*, white willow bark*, chamomile, coltsfoot, pennyroyal, rosemary, elder flower, thyme, marjoram, catnip, lavender, red clover.

IMMUNE SYSTEM HERBS: **Our Immune Power Formula**

Echinacea*, Siberian ginseng*, pau d' arco*, astragalus*, red clover, donq quai, ginger, orange peel, cat's claw, suma, grape seed extract, and ester C.

We've used immune support herbs for years, but today it's more important than ever. Perhaps, we've become more aware of what the immune system does. With this in mind, we put together an "Immune Power Formula."

Using this approach to health is smart and takes consistent use of immune boosting herbs and nutrition. You'll be very sick of hearing me say this, but here goes—bee pollen, bee pollen, bee pollen! The nutrition is the best and it supports the immune system. In addition, the following herbal combination is excellent. The herbs marked with the asterisk are main herbs.

LAXATIVE HERBS: **Our Easy Does It Formula**
Senna leaves*, licorice root *, anise seed*, blue malva*, red clover, peppermint, buckthorn bark, marshmallow root.

One cup of this each evening will keep you regular. But if you want to be regular while getting great nutrition, try bee pollen.

MONTHLY CRAMPS: **Ladies Monthly Tea**
Cramp bark*, rosemary*, pennyroyal*, thyme, and chamomile.

Drink this tea the day before your period to avoid problems. Pennyroyal increases the flow; cramp bark relieves cramping; rosemary has natural cortisone, and the other herbs are relaxing.

I recommend drinking a couple of cups a day or as needed. This formula can be capsuled and carried in your purse. Safe and effective.

MENOPAUSE, PMS AND OTHER FUN STUFF

During menopause, a woman's body slows down its production of hormones, resulting in mood changes, drying skin, hair loss, and other symptoms. After much reading and research, I discovered that plants have hormonal qualities. For centuries, women have been helping themselves with herbs and nutrition. However, it was a new concept for me that women could help themselves with PMS and menopause. The formula I put together includes balancers and cleansers for the female system. It also contains natural hormones like black cohosh and licorice for estrogen, and sarsaparilla for progesterone. Dong quai, a Chinese herb, is a balancer and contains B6. Our Chinese sisters have used this for centuries to stay younger longer.

Through the years, we have learned that this formula helps PMS, menopause, regulates the menses, and increases fertility. It depends on how you use it.

One cup daily (or 2 capsules) for 7 to 10 days before your period will help PMS. It helps with water retention, balances hormones and helps relieve cramps.

To regulate the menses, drink one cup daily (or take 2 capsules). If you can determine when your period should begin, start this regimen 21 to 24 days before. It may take a couple of months, but in most cases this regulates the period. For teenagers who have irregular cycles, this is a safe way to regulate the menses.

To help increase fertility, use this formula from the last day of your period until the day before the next cycle. A cup a day or 2 capsules will do it. This raises your hormone levels, making you more fertile. Also, to increase and improve the man's sperm, I suggest Siberian ginseng. We have seen this help many couples become pregnant.

Menopause is a wonderful passage. This formula provides you with the hormones you need. It helps manage hot flashes, mood swings, hair thinning, and dry skin. There is no reason that you can't enjoy getting older—old enough to be in charge of your life and young enough to have fun. Whether it is surgical or natural menopause, these herbs will make a difference. If you have no period, take it every day. If you still have a period, use it from the last day to the first. You may need to use more than we mentioned. Every woman is different. I take four capsules a day. Some women use more but most use three capsules per day. This equals two to three cups of tea.

We hear lots of positive comments from men on this formula. Many of the men folks coming in to the shop call "New Life Formula" happy pills.

New Life Formula

Red raspberry*, sarsaparilla*, Siberian ginseng*, scullcap*, licorice root*, black cohosh, yellow dock, lemon balm, dong quai, blessed thistle, angelica, nettle, wild yam, chaste tree berry and red clover.

In addition to the herbs in "New Life Formula," I would suggest vitamin E, bee pollen and royal jelly.

For those of you who just want the cleansing and balancing, eliminate sarsaparilla, black cohosh and licorice root.

MEN: **Men's complaints**

For years, there was an absence of men in our herb business. Wives and women friends talked to us about men's health. That has changed. It's wonderful to see men comfortable and ready to talk about physical problems. Of course, there are some physical complaints that men and women share. But those 'private' ones were seldom talked about. Impotence and prostrate problems were rarely mentioned. In the past twenty-five years, we have had an opportunity to help men with these.

IMPOTENCE: **Fountain of Youth**

Siberian ginseng*, sarsaparilla*, oat straw*, American ginseng*, saw palmetto*, burdock root*, red clover, alfalfa, celery seed, dandelion root, ginkgo, fo ti, propolis, horsetail, gotu kola, kelp, ginger and peppermint.

The "Fountain of Youth Formula" was put

together for our men customers because they felt slighted. Several men came in and complained that their wives were feeling "too good." They also needed something to help them age gracefully. After several weeks of study, I came up with the following formula: The tea or capsules help promote healthy hair, prostate, sex life, and the immune system. We recommend one to two cups a day or two to four capsules daily.

PROSTATE HEALTH: **Easy Flow**

Red clover*, burdock*, peppermint, horsetail*, saw palmetto*.

"Easy Flow Tea" can help with prostate cancer, which is a slow-growing form of the disease. I recommend two to three cups a day of "Easy Flow Tea." In addition, I suggest propolis and bee pollen for nutrition. This can also be used for prevention.

Men hesitate to talk about impotence. There is help! We recommend herbs that increase circulation and improve the health of the prostate. Also, I advise zinc (100 to 200 milligrams daily) and 800 units of vitamin E. Royal jelly and bee pollen are a must.

The men we have worked with report back to us—all systems go! For some, it takes a couple of months. For others, much less. These herbs also help improve overall health.

SKIN PROBLEMS: **Inside/Outside Tea**

Red clover*, oat straw*, sage*, elder flowers*, burdock, chamomile, lavender, peppermint, catnip, rosemary, and cinnamon powder for taste.

This tea consists of blood purifiers, nutritional herbs, and mild relaxants. I recommend three cups per day to drink and a stronger version to spray on trouble spots. Thus, the name of the formula! I suggest adding vitamin E to the spray and taking 800 IUs daily. You can also take B vitamins, brewers yeast or bee pollen, and extra zinc. (Never take zinc on an empty stomach).

Whether it's eczema or psoriasis, the formula and supplements make a difference. I prefer bee pollen to brewer's yeast and I suggest propolis. It helps the skin heal because it is an antibiotic. Propolis is available in tablet form and in cream. If you're serious about your skin, try them both.

Two of the herbs in this formula, rosemary and sage, have natural cortisone.

BLOOD SUGAR: **To Regulate and Lower**
For 17 years, we have been recommending one to two cups of blueberry leaf tea each day to control blood sugar. It's safe to do this with medication. The tea tastes good and regulates insulin. It's available in capsules.

Other herbs work with blueberry leaves or alone to lower sugar. Many folks have had success with yarrow (milfoil) and dandelion root. Blueberry is my first choice. Mix a tea with equal parts of each if you want to try cover all the bases.

BLOOD PRESSURE: **How to Lower and Control It**
Our "Dieter's Delight" has diuretics, which help lower blood pressure, and blueberry leaves to help regulate sugar as well as blood pressure. In addition to these two, I recommend vitamin E and cayenne red pepper because it helps lower blood pressure by improving circulation. I also use black cohosh and garlic.

You might feel that this is a lot to do to lower your

blood pressure. Because it takes more than one thing to create high blood pressure, it takes more than one thing to lower it.

When women reach the age of menopause, blood pressure can rise, so I recommend "New Life Tea Formula," as well.

WEIGHT LOSS: **Dieter's Delight** AND **FB2**

Everyone wants to lose weight, so we put together two formulas to help. "Dieter's Delight" has many herbal diuretics, nutritional herbs, and mild appetite suppressants. The herbs in Dieter's Delight have no stimulants and the taste is pleasant. We suggest drinking a cup or taking two capsules before meals.

Dieter's Delight

Alfalfa *, fennel seed*, parsley*, bladder wrack, blueberry leaves, corn silk, dandelion, kelp, uva ursi, Super Citrimax and L-Carnitine.

FB2

Guarana*, ephedra*(ma huang), white willow, Siberian ginseng*, green tea, gotu kola*, fennel*, bladder wrack*, kelp*, peppermint, ginger, parsley, chickweed and chromium.

The FB2 is one of the most popular blends we have. It is a stimulant. Guarana has lots of caffeine. Ephedra (ma huang) contains ephedrines and plant adrenaline. The formula has nutrients, appetite suppressants, and diuretics. We suggest 2 capsules before meals, not at bedtime.

STRESS: **The Sleep Tight Formula**

Chamomile*, hops*, catnip*, skullcap*, passion flower*, spearmint, lemon verbena, lavender and valerian extract. The valerian is not in the tea.

Stress creates an environment for illness. We blame everything on stress, but that is close to the truth. I recommend royal jelly and bee pollen. The rejuvenating qualities of royal jelly and the nutrition in bee pollen do the trick.

Why does pollen work for stress? The amino acids and B vitamins are major players. All in all, bee pollen supplies all the vitamins and minerals you need. It won't chase away the problems, but you will handle them differently. My customers tell me that they have lots of energy and a sense of well-being after taking bee pollen.

There are lots of safe herbal sedatives that help you sleep. In fact, many of them can be used daily. The Sleep Tight Formula relaxes you and still allows you to climb up the stairs to bed.

If you find that these sedative herbs are not strong enough, try additional valerian. Remember it does have an odor—capsules are the easiest way to take it.

Sinus Problems: **Pressure, Pain and Congestion**

Peppermint*, coltsfoot*, blue vervain*, mullein*, wild cherry bark*, rose hips*, sage*, thyme*, red clover, chamomile, yarrow, lemon peel, elder flower.

This "Sniffles Away Tea" helps open up the sinus passages and is a decongestant. It really helps with upper respiratory problems. It contains lots of vitamin C. You can drink as needed, or take it in capsule form for convenience.

I also recommend bee pollen to help with allergies. "Sniffles Away Tea" and natural antibiotics, goldenseal and propolis, helps relieve sinus problems.

SPORT TEA: **Increased Endurance and Energy**
  Siberian ginseng*, American ginseng*, Korean
  ginseng*, dandelion root*, ginger root*, nettles*,
  sarsaparilla*, caraway*, licorice root, ephedra, gotu
  kola, red clover, alfalfa, echinacea, and orange peel
  for flavor.

  This "#1 Son Sport Tea" is a really good-tasting
tea. It contains herbs for endurance and energy. A lot
of folks drink this when they have extra work to do.
Some of our customers call it the "power tea." Sport
formula and bee pollen will help you compete and
win!

TINNITUS: **Noise in the Ears**
This is a problem that is much more common than I
imagined. I recommend three cups a day for at least
two months. Folks report more energy and less illness. When you look at the herbs in the formula,
you'll understand why. The most important herb in
this blend is ginkgo. In fact, include ten times more
ginkgo than any other herb.

SERENITEA

Ginkgo*, Siberian ginseng*, sarsaparilla*, dandelion root*, astragalus*, ginger*, licorice root*, saw palmetto*, red clover, donq quai, black cohosh, American ginseng, gentian, gotu kola, peppermint for taste.

STOMACH PROBLEMS: **Indigestion, Upset Stomach, Colitis**

Peppermint*, catnip*, chamomile*, and slippery elm*.

If you drink a cup of this "Tummy Tea" formula before meals, you can avoid terrible indigestion. Today we recommend this combination for stomach flu, colic, ulcers, and nervous stomach. If you are dealing with digestive problems and/or colitis, add raspberry leaves and mullein.

CHRISTMAS CULINARY HERBS

Cooking was one of my least favorite things to do, until I discovered herbs. Between cooking the wild things in the meadow and seasoning "normal food" with herbs, the kitchen became a fun place. My sister, Linda, and I would have a "Euell Gibbons Day" dinner every so often. At first, the whole family would show up to partake. They became really suspicious of us after we served milkweed pods! Not only did we pass them off as okra, we encouraged eating seconds. Some of the family found that eating lots of milkweed pods can cause diarrhea. It was a learning experience for all of us. Linda and I still remember those days with a smile. I'm not recommending that you go to these extremes, but you can have fun in the kitchen.

Gifts from your kitchen or herb garden are really appreciated. A basket packed with your favorite herb seasonings, herb vinegar, a wooden spoon and a favorite recipe is a great gift.

Here are some of my favorite recipes:

Bouquet garni supreme: this is excellent in soups, breads, and stews. We always throw a bay leaf in the pot to add flavor.

4 teaspoons parsley; 1 teaspoon rosemary; 2 teaspoons sweet marjoram; 1 teaspoon celery seed; 4 teaspoons thyme; 1 teaspoon basil; and 2 tsp. savory.

Italian seasoning: this is delicious. Use in anything, even meatloaf.

5 teaspoons oregano; 3 teaspoons basil; 1 teaspoon thyme; ½ tsp. parley; ½ tsp. savory, ½ tsp. sweet marjoram.

Fish seasoning: whether your fish comes from the supermarket or a stream, this seasoning will compliment it:

2 tsp. lemon verbena; 3 teaspoons parsley; 2 teaspoons dill; 1 teaspoon basil; 1 teaspoon thyme.

Herb salt substitute: I keep this in a shaker on the stove. It goes in everything, except dessert. Mix these ingredients, put them in your blender, and grind to a fine powder. A little goes a long way.

5 teaspoons basil; 3 teaspoons savory; 1 teaspoon sage; 2 teaspoons celery seed; 1 teaspoon thyme; 2 teaspoons sweet marjoram; 4 teaspoons parsley; 1 teaspoon sassafras, ⅛ tsp. kelp.

Herb butter blend: mix 1 tbsp. of this in a ¼ pound of butter or marjoram, and serve. Get ready for compliments. I sometimes add fresh chopped chives. Try it on vegetables, in salads, and in soups.

A quick, delicious herb butter is made from equal parts of chives and thyme:

4 teaspoons thyme; 1 teaspoon parsley; 1 teaspoon sweet marjoram; 1 teaspoon summer savory; 1 teaspoon safflower; 1 teaspoon celery seed; ½ tsp. tarragon.

Easy French bread: the first bread I ever baked and it is fail proof. I had my parents to dinner and mom couldn't believe I baked it. She was sure I bought it. This bread makes a great gift. If you want it to be an herb bread, mix the herbs of choice in the dry ingredients. If you want a breakfast bread, add extra sugar (brown sugar is good) and ground cinnamon. Plop it on a cookie sheet like cookies and you have hamburger rolls. Roll it out and you have pizza crust. You don't even knead this bread!

To make it, dissolve 1 package of yeast in 1 cup of warm water. While waiting for this to start working mix the following ingredients: 1 cup of warm water;

4 cups of flour; 1 tbsp. Sugar; 1 teaspoon salt.

If you want a richer bread, replace part of the second cup of water with one egg. Add the yeast water and stir. The dough should be sticky. Add a little more flour if necessary. Cover the bowl with a towel and place in a warm place to rise. When it doubles in size, punch down and place in two greased, floured bread pans. Cover them with the towel and place in a warm place until double in size. Put the pans in a cold oven and turn to 400 degrees. Bake 30 minutes or until you can thump it and get a hollow sound. Remove from pans immediately and place on rack to cool.

• Herb vinegar: This is so easy. One of my favorite herb vinegars is made with Italian seasoning and brown apple cider vinegar. Add 1 gallon of vinegar to at least 1 ounce of dried Italian seasoning. Remove enough vinegar to get the herbs in and place in a warm or sunny spot. After three weeks or more, you can strain and bottle. While you wait for this to age, ask a beer drinker you know to save bottles for you. I usually go to the store and buy a couple of six packs. Choose the beer for the type of bottle, not taste.

Someone will eventually drink it. Your local hardware store should stock corks. Wash and scald the bottles. Strain the herbs out of the vinegar and bottle. I usually place a sprig of fresh herbs in the bottle. Tie on a ribbon and label your vinegar. This is an excellent gift. Check the prices for herb vinegar in the supermarket—they're expensive to buy, but easy and inexpensive to make.

Fragrance

If you have an herb or flower garden, you're bound to have leftovers. The best way to make use of these is to make potpourri. Most books make this sound pretty complicated. Here is a simple way to make potpourri. You can always get fancy later.

Start by drying petals, leaves, peels, moss, pinecones and spices, to mention a few. Anything goes when making a potpourri. Dry your materials in bundles, on a screen, or in a basket. It doesn't matter whether the dry materials smell good or not. We'll make them smell good! One of my first potpourris was called Grandmother's Garden. Someone asked me for a lilac potpourri. Lilacs don't hold their fragrance, so I came up with the following recipe:

Grandmother's Garden Potpourri

8 cups of green leaves (parsley and/or lemon balm);
2 handfuls of lavender (when available); 2 handfuls
of rose petals (when available); 6 cups of any color or
type of natural dried flower.

Put this in a plastic garbage bag and add 2 ounces of
orris root. The last step is to add two or three quarter
ounces of lilac fragrance oil. Shake it all up and
you've got it! Age it if you like, but if you need a
quick gift, package it and present it.

Most folks have access to mint so I thought a mint
potpourri would be useful. We call this one "Magical
Mint" because of the mugwort.

Magical Mint Potpourri

6 cups of dried mint leaves (peppermint, spearmint);
1 cup of mugwort; 2 cups of bergamot flowers and
leaves; 1 cup of dried moss; 2 cups of dried white flowers (pearly everlasting or perhaps lemon peel); 2 ounces
of orris root chips and 2 or 3 mint fragrance oils.

Mix it in a plastic bag so that the oil soaks into the

flowers and not your container. If you want this to be a Christmas potpourri, add cinnamon chips and dried orange peel. Dried geranium flowers add a nice touch of red.

Everyone loves rose potpourri. The flowers in this can vary, but you should have rose petals—just for looks. Patchouli compliments roses; that's why we add it.

Rose Potpourri

8 cups of rose petals or buds; 3 handfuls of marjoram; 5 handfuls of rosemary; 3 handfuls of patchouli; 4 handfuls of red flowers (poppy or hibiscus); 4 handfuls of blue malva; 3 handfuls of oak moss; 2 ounces of orris root; and 2 to 3 bottles of rose fragrance oil.

Spice Cupboard Potpourri

We have a Spice Cupboard potpourri that looks pretty and smells great. It doesn't need an oil, because it's all spices. You can simmer this one. Remember, if you don't have all the ingredients, use what you do have.

8 cups star anise; cup coriander seed; 2 cups broken

bay leaves; 2 cups whole allspice; 2 cups whole cloves; 5 whole nutmegs, broken; 2 cups whole ginger root; 1 cup orange peel; 1 cup lemon peel; 1 cup mustard seed; 1 cup fennel seed; 3 cups cinnamon chips; 2 cups hibiscus flowers; 2 ounces orris root chips.

If you have managed to collect and dry a grocery bag full of material, add 2 ounces of orris root and 2-3 fragrance oils of your choice. You can make a potpourri smell anyway you like. Fragrance is one of the many pleasures of your herb garden.

PETS AND HERBS

Over the years, I've had occasion to use many of my herb remedies on my pets. My dog, Cheyenne, takes our A&R formula so she could keep up with me on our daily walks. She takes bee pollen and garlic for her coat. The garlic helps keep fleas away.

I have 8 cats and they take bee pollen for nutrition. They don't always like it, but I'm bigger than they are! Cats have problems with urinary tract blockage and infection. I give my cats goldenseal tablets for this. It is antibiotic and has lots of vitamin C.

For ear infections or ear mites, I use garlic and goldenseal. To a cup of olive oil, I add one teaspoon of goldenseal and squeeze 4 garlic oil capsules into it. This works for people with ear infections, too. Just put several drops in the ear a couple times a day, or as needed.

For eye infections, goldenseal tea, strained twice, is wonderful. Goldenseal is gritty; this is the reason for straining the tea.

Fleas seem to be the biggest problem folks have with cats and dogs. Pennyroyal is the very best repellent herb. It doesn't kill fleas, it just repels them. You can take the dried herb and grind it to make your own flea powder; or you can sew together a long strip of cloth and fill with the herb. This makes a natural flea collar. You can take ¼ ounce of pennyroyal oil and add it to a quart of water to use as flea spray. Never use straight pennyroyal oil on your skin or your pet's skin. It can be deadly. It is quite safe, if you follow instructions.

The next problem is smell. No one likes to have a house that smells like dogs and cats. I take ¼ ounce of pennyroyal oil and use it in scrub water. It is very minty and smells great. You can use any fragrance oil in scrub water. I choose to use pennyroyal because it discourages fleas anywhere I scrub.

Just remember that you can use healing herbs for your pets. I will sometimes check with my vet, but she usually says go for it. The longer you work with herbs the more comfortable you will be with helping yourself and your pets.

Cosmetic Herbs

Herbs can condition your hair, moisturize your skin, shrink your pores and color your hair. What you put into your body is certainly reflected on the outside. With herbs, you can improve on that reflection.

Let's start at the top and work our way down the body. We've been using and selling these recipes for more than 17 years. Feel free to change and improve these recipes:

Herbs for Your Hair

To rinse your hair with herbs, make a strong tea and use it as the last rinse. Do not rinse it out. To make a strong cup of tea, use 1 tablespoon of herbs per cup of boiling water. After steeping, strain and use.

Hair rinse for brunettes: 3 teaspoons rosemary; 2 teaspoons black malva; 1 teaspoon sage; 1 teaspoon parsley; 1 teaspoon southernwood; ½ teaspoon nettles.

Hair rinse for blondes: 3 teaspoons calendula; 3 teaspoons chamomile; ½ teaspoon rosemary; ½ teaspoon parsley; ½ teaspoon nettles; 2 teaspoons lemon peel.

Herbs for Your Face

The herbs below can be used in two ways. Mix them together, put them in water, and steam your face, or put them in a quart of witch hazel and steep for 3 weeks in a warm place. Strain and you have a great skin freshener.

Strawberry leaves, roses petals, lemon grass, comfrey leaves, chamomile, elder flowers, horse-tail, sage, rosemary, and kelp.

I prefer using these herbs for a facial. Grind the herbs in your blender until fine. Mix the dry herbs with twice the amount of brewer's yeast. This facial tightens the skin and shrinks pores; it also heals and provides nutrition to your skin. Mix warm water with a couple of tablespoons of the facial mix until it has the consistency of a runny paste. Apply the mix to your face and let it dry. Leave it on for 20 minutes or more. At first it may feel uncomfortable. Wait a few minutes and it will be worth it. To remove, rinse off with warm water; you may have to use a wet cloth to remove all of it. If you don't use all of your herbal facial mix, save it in a covered container. It will keep in the refrigerator for a week.

Herbs for the Bath

An herb bath can be healing and relaxing. Take the herbs of choice and place them in a tea infuser or muslin bag. At this point, you have two choices. You can make a very strong cup of herb tea and add it to your bath, or you can draw very hot water into the tub and add the bag of herbs. Let it steep for 20 minutes and then add more water to make it comfortable. The two baths listed below are my favorites. Enjoy!

Slenderizing Rose Herb Bath

8 teaspoons rose petals; 1 teaspoon sweet marjoram; 2 teaspoons rosemary; 2 teaspoons lavender; 1 teaspoon elder flowers; 1 teaspoon chamomile; 1 teaspoon kelp; ¼ ounce rose fragrance oil.

Slenderizing Lemon Herb Bath

1 teaspoon elder flowers; 1 teaspoon comfrey leaves; 3 teaspoons lemon peel; 1 teaspoon marshmallow root; 1 teaspoon lemon grass; 1 teaspoon lemon verbena; 1 teaspoon lavender; ¼ teaspoon horsetail; 1 teaspoon kelp; ¼ ounce lemon fragrance oil.

About Sweet Annie

Ann Marie Wishard, lecturer, healer, author and herbalist, spent 33 years promoting well-being through common sense and nutrition. Her charismatic presentation of time-honored healing methods puts her in constant demand for television and radio talk shows in the United States and Canada. She also runs Sweet Annie Herbs, a small group of women dedicated to herbs and their beneficial properties. Ann Marie formulated over 18 natural blends to help heal specific ailments and maintain health. Her knowledge, research, integrity, and talent bring credibility to the herb business. She lives in Central Pennsylvania with a German shepherd and 8 cats. For more information on Sweet Annie Herbs, look up www.sweetannie.com. The phone number is 1-800-995-4372.

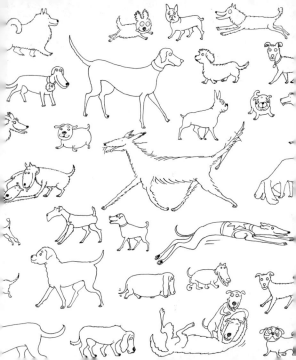

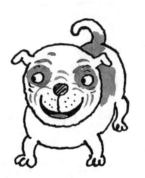